Metatextbook of Medicine

2011 subcollection of
2500 didactic
free medical review articles
a bibliography with
pmid numbers for Pubmed

To those
who in their everyday practice
thrive to translate
the science of biology
into
the art of medicine

To those
in need of an
inspiration
what they could, what they should
learn and enjoy
to
help mankind out of the trouble of
uncertaincity

To those who
deserve their lives
to
help their patients in the operating theatre
in the laboratories
on the computers
with any means of
humanity, gift and knowledge

This is a small selected bibliography of about 2.500 references to free medical review articles which have been selected because they are of interest to pupils, students and established healthcare professionals to work as the first scientific review articles they ever read, to be a source of inspiration of where-to-go and what-to-do, and to be some self-admistered CME load to learn what is going on out there.

It is a subcollection of my Metatextbook-of-Medicine on http://www.kidney.de, which originally shows 75.000 references to free medical review articles, which are tagged to 13.000 concepts and single-term items to cover all aspects of medicine and the life sciences.

While tagging references 30.000 up to 75.000, I specifically selected these few papers for inclusion of a subcollection serving those who want to be inspired by a bibliography rather than to select a random concept of 13.000 and to start from there - those professional people with essentially no knowledge on the cell cycle, on optical imaging, on running a clinical trial, on basic laboratory methodology, on treating cancer or the vasculitides - and indeed, the pupil as well as the senior physician will be enlightened by the material I referred to.

Nobody can be of current knowledge on the things out of his immediate scope, but indeed, he or she should have an approach to accessing a hot spot projection out of the whole literature.

Today, it needs one weeks time from formulating a search strategy for a literature database like pubmed and having collected all the papers regarded as relevant to the topic choosen. Today, the smallest ideas give 4 folders of papers, if retrieval was run with sensitive roc.

Since it is not possible to apply this approach beyond single highly-targeted questions to keep up with the ideas around, I designed the whole Metatextbook as "the review collection for wikipedia" - the spirit of an encyclopedia which is devoid of any own textual contents but which refers to a multitude of barrier-free accessible originally published review articles to introduce users into a topic.

I started the first 30.000 items on 3.000 topics on a default wikipedia collector and migrated into an unidirectional system of stable bibliographies which got published in early 2012 at about 60.000 items in 10.000 topics.

As shown above, this special, small subcollection of random sorted papers with the appeal of showing very interesting things is like carving out Proc-Natl-Acad-Sci-U-S-A from the wealth of 35M papers published in the life sciences, and it is reminiscent of going-copying in my early 90's when starting my studies in human medicine.

My readers (better, those of the authors whose work I have simply tagged and brought into focus) will enjoy having access to this small collection. You will decide whether my approach of giving you some marvellous but random stuff is something like an advent calendar, out of 24 items given, you will like one, so you have 100 little doors to open and look behind...

Winter 2012/2013 Ossip Groth

Simple advice how to use this resource:

Copypaste the PMID number (these 8 numbers in [bracketts] left-to the citation) into PubMed at http://www.ncbi.nih.nlm.gov/pubmed   (a.k.a. www.pubmed.org which redirects.)

Use this webpage http://www.kidney.de/MedlinePMID.php if PubMed does not locate a free pdf to the selected article.

Have a look at http://www.kidney.de/wiki/index.php?title=Mtbhelp %3AMetatextbook_Help_Page to learn more on the medical webresources which I have setup.

2009
1
Drug targets for traumatic brain injury from poly(ADP-ribose)polymerase pathway modulation.
[19371326] Br J Pharmacol 157(5):695-704 (2009)

2009
2
Therapeutic antibodies: successes, limitations and hopes for the future.
[19459844] Br J Pharmacol 157(2):220-33 (2009)

2009
3
Vitamin C: update on physiology and pharmacology.
[19508394] Br J Pharmacol 157(7):1097-110 (2009)

2008
4
A neuropeptide-centric view of psychostimulant addiction.
[18414383] Br J Pharmacol 154(2):343-57 (2008)

2008
5
Adenosine A2A receptor antagonists: blockade of adenosinergic effects and T regulatory cells.
[18311159] Br J Pharmacol 153 Suppl 1(-):S457-64 (2008)

2008
6
Proteinases and signalling: pathophysiological and therapeutic implications via PARs and more.
[18059329] Br J Pharmacol 153 Suppl 1(-):S263-82 (2008)

2008
7
Pharmacological approaches to acute ischaemic stroke: reperfusion certainly, neuroprotection possibly.
[18059324] Br J Pharmacol 153 Suppl 1(-):S325-38 (2008)

2008
8
Intracellular machinery for the transport of AMPA receptors.
[18026130] Br J Pharmacol 153 Suppl 1(-):S35-43 (2008)

2008
9
Fibroblasts as novel therapeutic targets in chronic inflammation.
[17965753] Br J Pharmacol 153 Suppl 1(-):S241-6 (2008)

2008
10
Cellular and molecular mechanisms responsible for the action of testosterone on human skeletal muscle. A basis for illegal performance enhancement.
[18414389] Br J Pharmacol 154(3):522-8 (2008)

2008
11
Asthma from a pharmacogenomic point of view.
[18311188] Br J Pharmacol 153(8):1602-14 (2008)

2008
12
Regulation of haeme oxygenase-1 for treatment of neuroinflammation and brain disorders.
[18794892] Br J Pharmacol 155(5):623-40 (2008)

2009
13
Protease-activated receptors and prostaglandins in inflammatory lung disease.
[19845685] Br J Pharmacol 158(4):1017-33 (2009)

2009
14
Exploiting the Annexin A1 pathway for the development of novel anti-inflammatory therapeutics.
[19845684] Br J Pharmacol 158(4):936-46 (2009)

2009
15
Mediators and receptors in the resolution of inflammation: drug targeting opportunities.
[19845683] Br J Pharmacol 158(4):933-5 (2009)

2009
16
Subtype-selective targeting of voltage-gated sodium channels.
[19845672] Br J Pharmacol 158(6):1413-25 (2009)

2009
17
Lipoxins: resolutionary road.
[19785661] Br J Pharmacol 158(4):947-59 (2009)

2009
18
Cyclin-dependent kinase inhibitor drugs as potential novel anti-inflammatory and pro-resolution agents.
[19775281] Br J Pharmacol 158(4):1004-16 (2009)

2009
19
Arginase: an emerging key player in the mammalian immune system.
[19764983] Br J Pharmacol 158(3):638-51 (2009)

2009
20
Prostanoid receptor antagonists: development strategies and therapeutic applications.
[19624532] Br J Pharmacol 158(1):104-45 (2009)

2009
21
Resolvins and protectins: mediating solutions to inflammation.
[19594757] Br J Pharmacol 158(4):960-71 (2009)

2009
22
Physical methods of nucleic acid transfer: general concepts and applications.
[19154421] Br J Pharmacol 157(2):207-19 (2009)

2008
23
Physiology and pharmacology of alcohol: the imidazobenzodiazepine alcohol antagonist site on subtypes of GABAA receptors as an opportunity for drug development?
[18278063] Br J Pharmacol 154(2):288-98 (2008)

2008
24
Plasmid encoded antibiotic resistance: acquisition and transfer of antibiotic resistance genes in bacteria.
[18193080] Br J Pharmacol 153 Suppl 1(-):S347-57 (2008)

2008
25
Prostamides (prostaglandin-ethanolamides) and their pharmacology.
[17721551] Br J Pharmacol 153(3):410-9 (2008)

2002
26
The developing relationship between receptor-operated and store-operated calcium channels in smooth muscle.
[11786473] Br J Pharmacol 135(1):1-13 (2002)

2010
27
Bimolecular fluorescence complementation: lighting up seven transmembrane domain receptor signalling networks.
[20015298] Br J Pharmacol 159(4):738-50 (2010)

2007
28
Chemogenomic approaches to rational drug design.
[17533416] Br J Pharmacol 152(1):38-52 (2007)

2007
29
Origin and evolution of high throughput screening.
[17603542] Br J Pharmacol 152(1):53-61 (2007)

2011
30
Endothelin.
[20848158] Cell Mol Life Sci 68(2):195-203 (2011)

2010
31
Mobile genetic elements of Staphylococcus aureus.
[20668911] Cell Mol Life Sci 67(18):3057-71 (2010)

2010
32
Post-transcriptional control during chronic inflammation and cancer: a focus on AU-rich elements.
[20495997] Cell Mol Life Sci 67(17):2937-55 (2010)

2010
33
Basement membrane components are key players in specialized extracellular matrices.
[20428923] Cell Mol Life Sci 67(17):2879-95 (2010)

2010
34
Rab protein evolution and the history of the eukaryotic endomembrane system.
[20582450] Cell Mol Life Sci 67(20):3449-65 (2010)

2010
35
Systems microscopy approaches to understand cancer cell migration and metastasis.
[20556632] Cell Mol Life Sci 67(19):3219-40 (2010)

2010
36
Sensing the fuels: glucose and lipid signaling in the CNS controlling energy homeostasis.
[20549539] Cell Mol Life Sci 67(19):3255-73 (2010)

2010
37
Oxidative damage to RNA: mechanisms, consequences, and diseases.
[20148281] Cell Mol Life Sci 67(11):1817-29 (2010)

2011
38
Stable transmission of reversible modifications: maintenance of epigenetic information through the cell cycle.
[20799050] Cell Mol Life Sci 68(1):27-44 (2011)

2010
39   **Targeting poly(ADP-ribose) polymerase activity for cancer therapy.**
[20725763] Cell Mol Life Sci 67(21):3649-62 (2010)

2006
40   **The parvins.**
[16314921] Cell Mol Life Sci 63(1):25-35 (2006)

2006
41   **The intriguing prion disorders.**
[16927029] Cell Mol Life Sci 63(19-20):2342-51 (2006)

2010
42   **Advanced optical imaging in living embryos.**
[20614161] Cell Mol Life Sci 67(20):3489-97 (2010)

2010
43   **Contrasting models for kinetochore microtubule attachment in mammalian cells.**
[20336345] Cell Mol Life Sci 67(13):2163-72 (2010)

2010
44   **Centrioles: active players or passengers during mitosis?**
[20300952] Cell Mol Life Sci 67(13):2173-94 (2010)

2010
45   **Finding the middle ground: how kinetochores power chromosome congression.**
[20232224] Cell Mol Life Sci 67(13):2145-61 (2010)

2010
46   **Mitotic force generators and chromosome segregation.**
[20221784] Cell Mol Life Sci 67(13):2231-50 (2010)

2011
47   **Genomic revelations of a mutualism: the pea aphid and its obligate bacterial symbiont.**
[21390549] Cell Mol Life Sci 68(8):1297-309 (2011)

2011
48   **Subcellular trafficking of the substrate transporters GLUT4 and CD36 in cardiomyocytes.**
[21547502] Cell Mol Life Sci 68(15):2525-38 (2011)

2011
49   **Membrane vesicles, current state-of-the-art: emerging role of extracellular vesicles.**
[21560073] Cell Mol Life Sci 68(16):2667-88 (2011)

2011
50   **Protecting the boundary: the sentinel role of host defense peptides in the skin.**
[21573782] Cell Mol Life Sci 68(13):2189-99 (2011)

2011
51   **SecA, a remarkable nanomachine.**
[21479870] Cell Mol Life Sci 68(12):2053-66 (2011)

2011
52   **The role of the proteasome in the generation of MHC class I ligands and immune responses.**
[21387144] Cell Mol Life Sci 68(9):1491-502 (2011)

2011
53   **Non-conventional sources of peptides presented by MHC class I.**
[21390547] Cell Mol Life Sci 68(9):1471-9 (2011)

2011
54   **The role of the precursor structure in the biogenesis of microRNA.**
[21607569] Cell Mol Life Sci 68(17):2859-71 (2011)

2011
55   **The STING pathway and regulation of innate immune signaling in response to DNA pathogens.**
[21161320] Cell Mol Life Sci 68(7):1157-65 (2011)

2011
56   **Advances in tenascin-C biology.**
[21818551] Cell Mol Life Sci 68(19):3175-99 (2011)

2011
57   **Mining electron density for functionally relevant protein polysterism in crystal structures.**
[21190057] Cell Mol Life Sci 68(11):1829-41 (2011)

2011
58   **Faithful chaperones.**
[21655914] Cell Mol Life Sci 68(20):3307-22 (2011)

2011   **Modes of Aβ² toxicity in Alzheimer's disease.**
59   [21706148] Cell Mol Life Sci 68(20):3359-75 (2011)

2011   **The gap gene network.**
60   [20927566] Cell Mol Life Sci 68(2):243-74 (2011)

2010   **Going up in flames: necrotic cell injury and inflammatory diseases.**
61   [20532807] Cell Mol Life Sci 67(19):3241-53 (2010)

2010   **Sexual reproduction in the Candida clade: cryptic cycles, diverse mechanisms, and alternative functions.**
62   [20552251] Cell Mol Life Sci 67(19):3275-85 (2010)

2011   **Chromosomal organization at the level of gene complexes.**
63   [21080026] Cell Mol Life Sci 68(6):977-90 (2011)

2010   **Bioinformatics and molecular modeling in glycobiology.**
64   [20364395] Cell Mol Life Sci 67(16):2749-72 (2010)

2010   **The elegans of spindle assembly.**
65   [20339898] Cell Mol Life Sci 67(13):2195-213 (2010)

2008   **Polyubiquitin chains: functions, structures, and mechanisms.**
66   [18438605] Cell Mol Life Sci 65(15):2397-406 (2008)

2008   **Amyloid beta-degrading cryptidases: insulin degrading enzyme, presequence peptidase, and neprilysin.**
67   [18470479] Cell Mol Life Sci 65(16):2574-85 (2008)

2010   **Helix insertion into bilayers and the evolution of membrane proteins.**
68   [20039094] Cell Mol Life Sci 67(7):1077-88 (2010)

2010   **Timing is everything: the regulation of type III secretion.**
69   [20043184] Cell Mol Life Sci 67(7):1065-75 (2010)

2010   **From protein sequences to 3D-structures and beyond: the example of the UniProt knowledgebase.**
70   [20043185] Cell Mol Life Sci 67(7):1049-64 (2010)

2010   **Platelets in defense against bacterial pathogens.**
71   [20013024] Cell Mol Life Sci 67(4):525-44 (2010)

2008   **Cell penetrating peptide inhibitors of nuclear factor-kappa B.**
72   [18668204] Cell Mol Life Sci 65(22):3564-91 (2008)

2010   **RNA-seq: from technology to biology.**
73   [19859660] Cell Mol Life Sci 67(4):569-79 (2010)

2010   **The molecular mechanisms of transition between mesenchymal and amoeboid invasiveness in tumor cells.**
74   [19707854] Cell Mol Life Sci 67(1):63-71 (2010)

2010   **Non-B DNA structure-induced genetic instability and evolution.**
75   [19727556] Cell Mol Life Sci 67(1):43-62 (2010)

2010   **Myosin motor function: the ins and outs of actin-based membrane protrusions.**
76   [20107861] Cell Mol Life Sci 67(8):1239-54 (2010)

2007   **Epigenetic control of nuclear architecture.**
77   [17221334] Cell Mol Life Sci 64(4):449-57 (2007)

2008
98
Role of HIV Gp41 mediated fusion/hemifusion in bystander apoptosis.
[18500445] Cell Mol Life Sci 65(20):3134-44 (2008)

2008
99
Methyl-CpG binding proteins: specialized transcriptional repressors or structural components of chromatin?
[18322651] Cell Mol Life Sci 65(10):1509-22 (2008)

2008
100
Substrate specificity of gamma-secretase and other intramembrane proteases.
[18239854] Cell Mol Life Sci 65(9):1311-34 (2008)

2008
101
Myosin V from head to tail.
[18239852] Cell Mol Life Sci 65(9):1378-89 (2008)

2008
102
Galanin impairs cognitive abilities in rodents: relevance to Alzheimer's disease.
[18500642] Cell Mol Life Sci 65(12):1836-41 (2008)

2008
103
Galanin in Alzheimer's disease: neuroinhibitory or neuroprotective?
[18500641] Cell Mol Life Sci 65(12):1842-53 (2008)

2008
104
Host cell manipulation by the human pathogen Toxoplasma gondii.
[18327664] Cell Mol Life Sci 65(12):1900-15 (2008)

2009
105
The dynamic nature of the bacterial cytoskeleton.
[19641848] Cell Mol Life Sci 66(20):3353-62 (2009)

2010
106
Cellular mechanisms regulating epithelial morphogenesis and cancer invasion.
[20832275] Curr Opin Cell Biol 22(5):640-50 (2010)

2010
107
Dynamic interplay between the collagen scaffold and tumor evolution.
[20822891] Curr Opin Cell Biol 22(5):697-706 (2010)

2010
108
3D shortcuts to gene regulation.
[20466532] Curr Opin Cell Biol 22(3):305-13 (2010)

2010
109
Decoding the function of nuclear long non-coding RNAs.
[20356723] Curr Opin Cell Biol 22(3):357-64 (2010)

2010
110
Down the rabbit hole of centromere assembly and dynamics.
[20303726] Curr Opin Cell Biol 22(3):392-402 (2010)

2010
111
Chromatin as a potential carrier of heritable information.
[20299197] Curr Opin Cell Biol 22(3):284-90 (2010)

2010
112
Quality and quantity control at the endoplasmic reticulum.
[20570125] Curr Opin Cell Biol 22(4):437-46 (2010)

2010
113
Cell biology of Ca2+-triggered exocytosis.
[20561775] Curr Opin Cell Biol 22(4):496-505 (2010)

2010
114
Manipulation of host membrane machinery by bacterial pathogens.
[20542678] Curr Opin Cell Biol 22(4):547-54 (2010)

2010
115
Transport at the recycling endosome.
[20541925] Curr Opin Cell Biol 22(4):528-34 (2010)

2010
116
Signaling endosomes: seeing is believing.
[20538448] Curr Opin Cell Biol 22(4):535-40 (2010)

2010
117
At the junction of SNARE and SM protein function.
[20471239] Curr Opin Cell Biol 22(4):488-95 (2010)

2010
118   **Regulation of coat assembly--sorting things out at the ER.**
            [20439155] Curr Opin Cell Biol 22(4):447-53 (2010)

2010
119   **Structure and mechanism in membrane trafficking.**
            [20418086] Curr Opin Cell Biol 22(4):454-60 (2010)

2010
120   **The ciliary membrane.**
            [20399632] Curr Opin Cell Biol 22(4):541-6 (2010)

2011   **Modern fluorescent proteins and imaging technologies to study gene expression, nuclear**
121   **localization, and dynamics.**
            [21242078] Curr Opin Cell Biol 23(3):310-7 (2011)

2011
122   **Endosomal signaling and cell migration.**
            [21546233] Curr Opin Cell Biol 23(5):615-20 (2011)

2011
123   **The role of adhesion energy in controlling cell-cell contacts.**
            [21807491] Curr Opin Cell Biol 23(5):508-14 (2011)

2010
124   **VE-cadherin: at the front, center, and sides of endothelial cell organization and function.**
            [20708398] Curr Opin Cell Biol 22(5):651-8 (2010)

2010
125   **Cell adhesion in regulation of asymmetric stem cell division.**
            [20724132] Curr Opin Cell Biol 22(5):605-10 (2010)

2010
126   **Conserved F-actin dynamics and force transmission at cell adhesions.**
            [20728328] Curr Opin Cell Biol 22(5):583-8 (2010)

2011
127   **Protein misfolding disorders and macroautophagy.**
            [21087849] Curr Opin Cell Biol 23(2):190-7 (2011)

2008
128   **Trans-cellular migration: cell-cell contacts get intimate.**
            [18595683] Curr Opin Cell Biol 20(5):533-40 (2008)

2008
129   **The killer's kiss: the many functions of NK cell immunological synapses.**
            [18639449] Curr Opin Cell Biol 20(5):597-605 (2008)

2008
130   **Collagen fibrillogenesis: fibronectin, integrins, and minor collagens as organizers and nucleators.**
            [18640274] Curr Opin Cell Biol 20(5):495-501 (2008)

2004
131   **Regulation of matrix biology by matrix metalloproteinases.**
            [15363807] Curr Opin Cell Biol 16(5):558-64 (2004)

2009
132   **Making the Auroras glow: regulation of Aurora A and B kinase function by interacting proteins.**
            [19836940] Curr Opin Cell Biol 21(6):796-805 (2009)

2010
133   **TOR-dependent control of autophagy: biting the hand that feeds.**
            [20006481] Curr Opin Cell Biol 22(2):157-68 (2010)

2010
134   **Mammalian autophagy: core molecular machinery and signaling regulation.**
            [20034776] Curr Opin Cell Biol 22(2):124-31 (2010)

2010
135   **Mechanics of cytokinesis in eukaryotes.**
            [20031383] Curr Opin Cell Biol 22(1):50-6 (2010)

2010
136   **Cytoprotective roles for autophagy.**
            [20045304] Curr Opin Cell Biol 22(2):206-11 (2010)

2010
137   **Role of autophagy in suppression of inflammation and cancer.**
            [20056400] Curr Opin Cell Biol 22(2):212-7 (2010)

2010 **Autophagy in infection.**
138 [20116986] Curr Opin Cell Biol 22(2):252-62 (2010)

2010 **Necroptosis as an alternative form of programmed cell death.**
139 [20045303] Curr Opin Cell Biol 22(2):263-8 (2010)

2007 **Lysosome-related organelles: driving post-Golgi compartments into specialisation.**
140 [17628466] Curr Opin Cell Biol 19(4):394-401 (2007)

2007 **Lipids and lipid modifications in the regulation of membrane traffic.**
141 [17651957] Curr Opin Cell Biol 19(4):426-35 (2007)

2007 **Dysferlin and muscle membrane repair.**
142 [17662592] Curr Opin Cell Biol 19(4):409-16 (2007)

2007 **Cell adhesion molecules and actin cytoskeleton at immune synapses and kinapses.**
143 [17923403] Curr Opin Cell Biol 19(5):529-33 (2007)

2007 **Structure and mechanics of integrin-based cell adhesion.**
144 [17928215] Curr Opin Cell Biol 19(5):495-507 (2007)

2007 **Making and breaking contacts: the cellular biology of cadherin regulation.**
145 [17935963] Curr Opin Cell Biol 19(5):508-14 (2007)

2007 **Catenins: playing both sides of the synapse.**
146 [17936606] Curr Opin Cell Biol 19(5):551-6 (2007)

2007 **Desmosomes from a structural perspective.**
147 [17945476] Curr Opin Cell Biol 19(5):565-71 (2007)

2007 **Mechanisms controlling cell cycle exit upon terminal differentiation.**
148 [18035529] Curr Opin Cell Biol 19(6):697-704 (2007)

2007 **Receptor tyrosine kinases: mechanisms of activation and signaling.**
149 [17306972] Curr Opin Cell Biol 19(2):117-23 (2007)

2008 **Centrioles: some self-assembly required.**
150 [18840522] Curr Opin Cell Biol 20(6):688-93 (2008)

2008 **The quality control of MHC class I peptide loading.**
151 [18926908] Curr Opin Cell Biol 20(6):624-31 (2008)

2009 **Probing the macromolecular organization of cells by electron tomography.**
152 [19185480] Curr Opin Cell Biol 21(1):89-96 (2009)

2009 **Centriole evolution.**
153 [19196504] Curr Opin Cell Biol 21(1):14-9 (2009)

2009 **Polysomes, P bodies and stress granules: states and fates of eukaryotic mRNAs.**
154 [19394210] Curr Opin Cell Biol 21(3):403-8 (2009)

2009 **Substrate-specific mediators of ER associated degradation (ERAD).**
155 [19443192] Curr Opin Cell Biol 21(4):516-21 (2009)

2009 **Peripheral ER structure and function.**
156 [19447593] Curr Opin Cell Biol 21(4):596-602 (2009)

2009 **The exocyst complex in polarized exocytosis.**
157 [19473826] Curr Opin Cell Biol 21(4):537-42 (2009)

2009
158 The basal initiation machinery: beyond the general transcription factors.
[19411170] Curr Opin Cell Biol 21(3):344-51 (2009)

2009
159 Turnover of organelles by autophagy in yeast.
[19515549] Curr Opin Cell Biol 21(4):522-30 (2009)

2009
160 Nuclear pore complex biogenesis.
[19524430] Curr Opin Cell Biol 21(4):603-12 (2009)

2009
161 Extracellular microfibrils: contextual platforms for TGFbeta and BMP signaling.
[19525102] Curr Opin Cell Biol 21(5):616-22 (2009)

2009
162 The signaling mechanisms of syndecan heparan sulfate proteoglycans.
[19535238] Curr Opin Cell Biol 21(5):662-9 (2009)

2008
163 Transcriptional control by PARP-1: chromatin modulation, enhancer-binding, coregulation, and insulation.
[18450439] Curr Opin Cell Biol 20(3):294-302 (2008)

2008
164 Mechanisms and cellular roles of local protein synthesis in mammalian cells.
[18378131] Curr Opin Cell Biol 20(2):144-9 (2008)

2008
165 Wnt/beta-catenin signaling: new (and old) players and new insights.
[18339531] Curr Opin Cell Biol 20(2):119-25 (2008)

2008
166 The multi-tasking P-TEFb complex.
[18513937] Curr Opin Cell Biol 20(3):334-40 (2008)

2008
167 New twists in X-chromosome inactivation.
[18508252] Curr Opin Cell Biol 20(3):349-55 (2008)

2008
168 Transcriptional targets of sirtuins in the coordination of mammalian physiology.
[18468877] Curr Opin Cell Biol 20(3):303-9 (2008)

2008
169 Multivesicular bodies: co-ordinated progression to maturity.
[18502633] Curr Opin Cell Biol 20(4):408-14 (2008)

2008
170 Retromer.
[18472259] Curr Opin Cell Biol 20(4):427-36 (2008)

2009
171 Polarity proteins regulate mammalian cell-cell junctions and cancer pathogenesis.
[19729289] Curr Opin Cell Biol 21(5):694-700 (2009)

2009
172 Cellular and nuclear degradation during apoptosis.
[19781927] Curr Opin Cell Biol 21(6):900-12 (2009)

2009
173 Mitochondrial reactive oxygen species regulate hypoxic signaling.
[19781926] Curr Opin Cell Biol 21(6):894-9 (2009)

2009
174 Assembly of ribosomes and spliceosomes: complex ribonucleoprotein machines.
[19167202] Curr Opin Cell Biol 21(1):109-18 (2009)

2009
175 Regulation of peroxisome dynamics.
[19188056] Curr Opin Cell Biol 21(1):119-26 (2009)

2008
176 Cargo transport: molecular motors navigate a complex cytoskeleton.
[18226515] Curr Opin Cell Biol 20(1):41-7 (2008)

2008
177 ESCRT complexes and the biogenesis of multivesicular bodies.
[18222686] Curr Opin Cell Biol 20(1):4-11 (2008)

2008   **Cilia orientation and the fluid mechanics of development.**
178   [18194854] Curr Opin Cell Biol 20(1):48-52 (2008)

2008   **Regulation of membrane trafficking in polarized epithelial cells.**
179   [18282697] Curr Opin Cell Biol 20(2):208-13 (2008)

2010   **A look at autoimmunity and inflammation in the eye.**
180   [20811163] J Clin Invest 120(9):3073-83 (2010)

2010   **How cortical neurons help us see: visual recognition in the human brain.**
181   [20811161] J Clin Invest 120(9):3054-63 (2010)

2010   **Retinopathy of prematurity: understanding ischemic retinal vasculopathies at an extreme of life.**
182   [20811158] J Clin Invest 120(9):3022-32 (2010)

2010   **Uric acid transport and disease.**
183   [20516647] J Clin Invest 120(6):1791-9 (2010)

2010   **From skin cells to hepatocytes: advances in application of iPS cell technology.**
184   [20739747] J Clin Invest 120(9):3102-5 (2010)

2011   **Cytomegalovirus: pathogen, paradigm, and puzzle.**
185   [21659716] J Clin Invest 121(5):1673-80 (2011)

2011   **Cellular pathophysiology of ischemic acute kidney injury.**
186   [22045571] J Clin Invest 121(11):4210-21 (2011)

2011   **Insight into the heterogeneity of breast cancer through next-generation sequencing.**
187   [21965338] J Clin Invest 121(10):3810-8 (2011)

2011   **Therapeutic strategies for the clinical blockade of IL-6/gp130 signaling.**
188   [21881215] J Clin Invest 121(9):3375-83 (2011)

2011   **Oxidized CaMKII: a "heart stopper" for the sinus node?**
189   [21785211] J Clin Invest 121(8):2975-7 (2011)

2011   **Recent advances in the molecular pathophysiology of atrial fibrillation.**
190   [21804195] J Clin Invest 121(8):2955-68 (2011)

2011   **The three R's of lung health and disease: repair, remodeling, and regeneration.**
191   [21633173] J Clin Invest 121(6):2065-73 (2011)

2011   **Adipose tissue remodeling and obesity.**
192   [21633177] J Clin Invest 121(6):2094-101 (2011)

2011   **The role of lipid droplets in metabolic disease in rodents and humans.**
193   [21633178] J Clin Invest 121(6):2102-10 (2011)

2010   **Pain as a channelopathy.**
194   [21041956] J Clin Invest 120(11):3745-52 (2010)

2010   **The discovery and development of analgesics: new mechanisms, new modalities.**
195   [21041957] J Clin Invest 120(11):3753-9 (2010)

2010   **Nociceptors: the sensors of the pain pathway.**
196   [21041958] J Clin Invest 120(11):3760-72 (2010)

2010   **Central modulation of pain.**
197   [21041960] J Clin Invest 120(11):3779-87 (2010)

2010 How we are born.
198 [20364092] J Clin Invest 120(4):952-5 (2010)

2010 The key role of vitamin A in spermatogenesis.
199 [20364093] J Clin Invest 120(4):956-62 (2010)

2010 The ovary: basic biology and clinical implications.
200 [20364094] J Clin Invest 120(4):963-72 (2010)

2010 Portrait of an oocyte: our obscure origin.
201 [20364095] J Clin Invest 120(4):973-83 (2010)

2010 Fertilization: a sperm's journey to and interaction with the oocyte.
202 [20364096] J Clin Invest 120(4):984-94 (2010)

2010 Making the blastocyst: lessons from the mouse.
203 [20364097] J Clin Invest 120(4):995-1003 (2010)

2005 Mitochondria: pharmacological manipulation of cell death.
204 [16200197] J Clin Invest 115(10):2640-7 (2005)

2005 Minding the gaps to promote thrombus growth and stability.
205 [16322784] J Clin Invest 115(12):3385-92 (2005)

2004 Salt handling and hypertension.
206 [15085183] J Clin Invest 113(8):1075-81 (2004)

2004 When cells get stressed: an integrative view of cellular senescence.
207 [14702100] J Clin Invest 113(1):8-13 (2004)

2003 Interspecies communication in bacteria.
208 [14597753] J Clin Invest 112(9):1291-9 (2003)

2003 The enigma of sepsis.
209 [12925683] J Clin Invest 112(4):460-7 (2003)

2003 Messenger RNA reprogramming by spliceosome-mediated RNA trans-splicing.
210 [12925685] J Clin Invest 112(4):474-80 (2003)

2003 The organization and consequences of eicosanoid signaling.
211 [12697726] J Clin Invest 111(8):1107-13 (2003)

2003 Endogenous generation of reactive oxidants and electrophiles and their reactions with DNA and
212 protein.
[12618510] J Clin Invest 111(5):583-93 (2003)

2003 Specificity of a third kind: reactive oxygen and nitrogen intermediates in cell signaling.
213 [12639979] J Clin Invest 111(6):769-78 (2003)

2008 Macrophage diversity in renal injury and repair.
214 [18982158] J Clin Invest 118(11):3522-30 (2008)

2010 Enabling stem cell therapies through synthetic stem cell-niche engineering.
215 [20051637] J Clin Invest 120(1):60-70 (2010)

2010 The therapeutic promise of the cancer stem cell concept.
216 [20051635] J Clin Invest 120(1):41-50 (2010)

2009 Targeted electrode-based modulation of neural circuits for depression.
217 [19339763] J Clin Invest 119(4):717-25 (2009)

2008   **The spread, treatment, and prevention of HIV-1: evolution of a global pandemic.**
218   [18382737] J Clin Invest 118(4):1244-54 (2008)

2008   **The anticancer immune response: indispensable for therapeutic success?**
219   [18523649] J Clin Invest 118(6):1991-2001 (2008)

2009   **Coadaptation of Helicobacter pylori and humans: ancient history, modern implications.**
220   [19729845] J Clin Invest 119(9):2475-87 (2009)

2009   **Intermediate filaments: primary determinants of cell architecture and plasticity.**
221   [19587452] J Clin Invest 119(7):1772-83 (2009)

2009   **"IF-pathies": a broad spectrum of intermediate filament-associated diseases.**
222   [19587450] J Clin Invest 119(7):1756-62 (2009)

2009   **Introducing intermediate filaments: from discovery to disease.**
223   [19587451] J Clin Invest 119(7):1763-71 (2009)

2010   **Teratogenic mechanisms of medical drugs.**
224   [20061329] Hum Reprod Update 16(4):378-94 (2010)

2010   **An immunological insight into the origins of pre-eclampsia.**
225   [20388637] Hum Reprod Update 16(5):510-24 (2010)

2002   **Current concepts in preimplantation genetic diagnosis (PGD): a molecular biologist's view.**
226   [11866237] Hum Reprod Update 8(1):11-20 (2002)

2002   **The molecular basis of sperm-oocyte membrane interactions during mammalian fertilization.**
227   [12206465] Hum Reprod Update 8(4):297-311 (2002)

2002   **The molecular foundations of the maternal to zygotic transition in the preimplantation embryo.**
228   [12206467] Hum Reprod Update 8(4):323-31 (2002)

2002   **Role of acrosomal matrix proteases in sperm-zona pellucida interactions.**
229   [12398221] Hum Reprod Update 8(5):405-12 (2002)

2011   **Maternal smoking in pregnancy and birth defects: a systematic review based on 173 687 malformed cases and 11.7 million controls.**
230   [21747128] Hum Reprod Update 17(5):589-604 (2011)

2010   **Fertility preservation in girls during childhood: is it feasible, efficient and safe and to whom should it be proposed?**
231   [20462941] Hum Reprod Update 16(6):617-30 (2010)

2010   **World Health Organization reference values for human semen characteristics.**
232   [19934213] Hum Reprod Update 16(3):231-45 (2010)

2008   **Control of hyperactivation in sperm.**
233   [18653675] Hum Reprod Update 14(6):647-57 (2008)

2004   **Cytoplasmic transfer in oocytes: biochemical aspects.**
234   [15140871] Hum Reprod Update 10(3):241-50 (2004)

2004   **Fertility preservation in female patients.**
235   [15140872] Hum Reprod Update 10(3):251-66 (2004)

2004   **Meiotic and mitotic nondisjunction: lessons from preimplantation genetic diagnosis.**
236   [15319376] Hum Reprod Update 10(5):401-7 (2004)

2004
237
Preserving the reproductive potential of men and boys with cancer: current concepts and future prospects.
[15319377] Hum Reprod Update 10(6):525-32 (2004)

2004
238
Syncytin: the major regulator of trophoblast fusion? Recent developments and hypotheses on its action.
[15333590] Hum Reprod Update 10(6):487-96 (2004)

2005
239
Cell-free fetal DNA in maternal blood: kinetics, source and structure.
[15569699] Hum Reprod Update 11(1):59-67 (2005)

2005
240
The chromosomal analysis of human oocytes. An overview of established procedures.
[15569701] Hum Reprod Update 11(1):15-32 (2005)

2005
241
Preimplantation genetic diagnosis and chromosome analysis of blastomeres using comparative genomic hybridization.
[15569702] Hum Reprod Update 11(1):33-41 (2005)

2003
242
The biological basis of non-invasive strategies for selection of human oocytes and embryos.
[12859045] Hum Reprod Update 9(3):237-49 (2003)

2003
243
Selection based on morphological assessment of oocytes and embryos at different stages of preimplantation development: a review.
[12859046] Hum Reprod Update 9(3):251-62 (2003)

2003
244
Review of clinical course and treatment of ovarian hyperstimulation syndrome (OHSS).
[12638783] Hum Reprod Update 9(1):77-96 (2003)

2010
245
Options for fertility preservation in prepubertal boys.
[20047952] Hum Reprod Update 16(3):312-28 (2010)

2007
246
Which is the best sperm retrieval technique for non-obstructive azoospermia? A systematic review.
[17895238] Hum Reprod Update 13(6):539-49 (2007)

2007
247
Altered protamine expression and diminished spermatogenesis: what is the link?
[17208950] Hum Reprod Update 13(3):313-27 (2007)

2007
248
Molecular mechanisms of ovulation: co-ordination through the cumulus complex.
[17242016] Hum Reprod Update 13(3):289-312 (2007)

2007
249
Mid-trimester induced abortion: a review.
[17050523] Hum Reprod Update 13(1):37-52 (2007)

2005
250
Apoptosis in the ovary: molecular mechanisms.
[15705959] Hum Reprod Update 11(2):162-77 (2005)

2005
251
The role of proteins of the transforming growth factor-beta superfamily in the intraovarian regulation of follicular development.
[15705960] Hum Reprod Update 11(2):143-60 (2005)

2005
252
Biological basis for human capacitation.
[15817522] Hum Reprod Update 11(3):205-14 (2005)

2005
253
Efforts to create an artificial testis: culture systems of male germ cells under biochemical conditions resembling the seminiferous tubular biochemical environment.
[15817525] Hum Reprod Update 11(3):229-59 (2005)

2008
254
Effects of environmental and occupational pesticide exposure on human sperm: a systematic review.
[18281240] Hum Reprod Update 14(3):233-42 (2008)

2008 255	**Impact of endocrine disruptor chemicals in gynaecology.** [18070835] Hum Reprod Update 14(1):59-72 (2008)

| 2008
256 | **Dealing with uncertainties: ethics of prenatal diagnosis and preimplantation genetic diagnosis to prevent mitochondrial disorders.**
[18056133] Hum Reprod Update 14(1):83-94 (2008) |

| 2008
257 | **Meiosis in oocytes: predisposition to aneuploidy and its increased incidence with age.**
[18084010] Hum Reprod Update 14(2):143-58 (2008) |

| 2006
258 | **The role and limits of a gradient based explanation of morphogenesis: a theoretical consideration.**
[16479501] Int J Dev Biol 50(2-3):333-40 (2006) |

| 2006
259 | **The natural variability of morphogenesis: a tool for exploring the mechanics of gastrulation movements in amphibian embryos.**
[16479499] Int J Dev Biol 50(2-3):315-22 (2006) |

| 2006
260 | **Morphodynamics of phyllotaxis.**
[16479495] Int J Dev Biol 50(2-3):277-87 (2006) |

| 2006
261 | **Mechanical control of tissue morphogenesis during embryological development.**
[16479493] Int J Dev Biol 50(2-3):255-66 (2006) |

| 2006
262 | **Mechanics in embryogenesis and embryonics: prime mover or epiphenomenon?**
[16479492] Int J Dev Biol 50(2-3):245-53 (2006) |

| 2006
263 | **Biophysical regulation during cardiac development and application to tissue engineering.**
[16479491] Int J Dev Biol 50(2-3):233-43 (2006) |

| 2006
264 | **Morphomechanics: goals, basic experiments and models.**
[16479477] Int J Dev Biol 50(2-3):81-92 (2006) |

| 2002
265 | **Vertebrate limb regeneration and the origin of limb stem cells.**
[12455626] Int J Dev Biol 46(7):887-96 (2002) |

| 2002
266 | **Limb muscle development.**
[12455628] Int J Dev Biol 46(7):905-14 (2002) |

| 2002
267 | **Signals regulating muscle formation in the limb during embryonic development.**
[12455629] Int J Dev Biol 46(7):915-25 (2002) |

| 2002
268 | **Wnt signalling during limb development.**
[12455630] Int J Dev Biol 46(7):927-36 (2002) |

| 2002
269 | **Human limb malformations; an approach to the molecular basis of development.**
[12455638] Int J Dev Biol 46(7):983-91 (2002) |

| 2002
270 | **Cnidarians as a model system for understanding evolution and regeneration.**
[11902686] Int J Dev Biol 46(1):39-48 (2002) |

| 2002
271 | **The genetic control of eye development and its implications for the evolution of the various eye-types.**
[11902689] Int J Dev Biol 46(1):65-73 (2002) |

| 2002
272 | **Conserved genetic mechanisms for embryonic brain patterning.**
[11902691] Int J Dev Biol 46(1):81-7 (2002) |

| 2002
273 | **Genetic studies define MAGUK proteins as regulators of epithelial cell polarity.**
[12141438] Int J Dev Biol 46(4):511-8 (2002) |

2002
274

Developmental basis of limb evolution.
[12455618] Int J Dev Biol 46(7):835-45 (2002)

2002
275

The progress zone model for specifying positional information.
[12455622] Int J Dev Biol 46(7):869-70 (2002)

2002
276

Programmed cell death in the developing limb.
[12455623] Int J Dev Biol 46(7):871-6 (2002)

2002
277

Interplay between the molecular signals that control vertebrate limb development.
[12455624] Int J Dev Biol 46(7):877-81 (2002)

2002
278

Retinoic acid and limb regeneration--a personal view.
[12455625] Int J Dev Biol 46(7):883-6 (2002)

2011
279

The role of pericytes in angiogenesis.
[21710434] Int J Dev Biol 55(3):261-8 (2011)

2011
280

The interplay between macrophages and angiogenesis in development, tissue injury and regeneration.
[21732273] Int J Dev Biol 55(4-5):495-503 (2011)

2004
281

Neurotrophic regulation of retinal ganglion cell synaptic connectivity: from axons and dendrites to synapses.
[15558485] Int J Dev Biol 48(8-9):947-56 (2004)

2004
282

New views on retinal axon development: a navigation guide.
[15558486] Int J Dev Biol 48(8-9):957-64 (2004)

2004
283

Retinal stem cells and regeneration.
[15558491] Int J Dev Biol 48(8-9):1003-14 (2004)

2004
284

Anterior segment development relevant to glaucoma.
[15558492] Int J Dev Biol 48(8-9):1015-29 (2004)

2004
285

Germinal tumor invasion and the role of the testicular stroma.
[15349829] Int J Dev Biol 48(5-6):545-57 (2004)

2005
286

Seed maturation: developing an intrusive phase to accomplish a quiescent state.
[16096971] Int J Dev Biol 49(5-6):645-51 (2005)

2005
287

The signal transducing photoreceptors of plants.
[16096972] Int J Dev Biol 49(5-6):653-64 (2005)

2005
288

Control of reproduction by Polycomb Group complexes in animals and plants.
[16096976] Int J Dev Biol 49(5-6):707-16 (2005)

2005
289

Sclerotome development and morphogenesis: when experimental embryology meets genetics.
[15906245] Int J Dev Biol 49(2-3):301-8 (2005)

2005
290

Historical perspectives on plant developmental biology.
[16096956] Int J Dev Biol 49(5-6):453-65 (2005)

2005
291

Balance between cell division and differentiation during plant development.
[16096957] Int J Dev Biol 49(5-6):467-77 (2005)

2005
292

Plant stem cell niches.
[16096958] Int J Dev Biol 49(5-6):479-89 (2005)

2005
293
Circadian clock signaling in Arabidopsis thaliana: from gene expression to physiology and development.
[16096959] Int J Dev Biol 49(5-6):491-500 (2005)

2005
294
Regulation of gene expression by light.
[16096960] Int J Dev Biol 49(5-6):501-11 (2005)

2005
295
Regulation of phyllotaxis.
[16096963] Int J Dev Biol 49(5-6):539-46 (2005)

2005
296
Leaf shape: genetic controls and environmental factors.
[16096964] Int J Dev Biol 49(5-6):547-55 (2005)

2005
297
Plastids unleashed: their development and their integration in plant development.
[16096965] Int J Dev Biol 49(5-6):557-77 (2005)

2005
298
Flowering: a time for integration.
[16096967] Int J Dev Biol 49(5-6):585-93 (2005)

2005
299
The making of gametes in higher plants.
[16096968] Int J Dev Biol 49(5-6):595-614 (2005)

2005
300
Flower and fruit development in Arabidopsis thaliana.
[16096970] Int J Dev Biol 49(5-6):633-43 (2005)

2003
301
Origin and evolution of endoderm and mesoderm.
[14756329] Int J Dev Biol 47(7-8):531-9 (2003)

2003
302
The origin and evolution of the nervous system.
[14756331] Int J Dev Biol 47(7-8):555-62 (2003)

2003
303
The Cambrian "explosion" of metazoans and molecular biology: would Darwin be satisfied?
[14756326] Int J Dev Biol 47(7-8):505-15 (2003)

2010
304
Primitive and definitive erythropoiesis in the yolk sac: a bird's eye view.
[20563984] Int J Dev Biol 54(6-7):1033-43 (2010)

2010
305
Primitive erythropoiesis in the mammalian embryo.
[20711979] Int J Dev Biol 54(6-7):1011-8 (2010)

2010
306
Embryonic origin of human hematopoiesis.
[20711983] Int J Dev Biol 54(6-7):1061-5 (2010)

2010
307
The Notch pathway in the developing hematopoietic system.
[20711994] Int J Dev Biol 54(6-7):1175-88 (2010)

2010
308
Structure and functions of powerful transactivators: VP16, MyoD and FoxA.
[21404180] Int J Dev Biol 54(11-12):1589-96 (2010)

2010
309
Improvement of mouse cloning using nuclear transfer-derived embryonic stem cells and/or histone deacetylase inhibitor.
[21404185] Int J Dev Biol 54(11-12):1641-8 (2010)

2010
310
The seminal work of Werner Risau in the study of the development of the vascular system.
[20209430] Int J Dev Biol 54(4):567-72 (2010)

2010
311
Molecular mechanisms controlling brain development: an overview of neuroepithelial secondary organizers.
[19876817] Int J Dev Biol 54(1):7-20 (2010)

2009   **Role of polycomb proteins Ring1A and Ring1B in the epigenetic regulation of gene expression.**
312   [19412891] Int J Dev Biol 53(2-3):355-70 (2009)

2009   **Function and specificity of Hox genes.**
313   [19247930] Int J Dev Biol 53(8-10):1404-19 (2009)

2009   **Segmentation, metamerism and the Cambrian explosion.**
314   [19247939] Int J Dev Biol 53(8-10):1305-16 (2009)

2007   **Establishment of a proneural field in the inner ear.**
315   [17891711] Int J Dev Biol 51(6-7):483-93 (2007)

2007   **Hindbrain signals in otic regionalization: walk on the wild side.**
316   [17891712] Int J Dev Biol 51(6-7):495-506 (2007)

2007   **Axial patterning in the developing vertebrate inner ear.**
317   [17891713] Int J Dev Biol 51(6-7):507-20 (2007)

2007   **Patterning and morphogenesis of the vertebrate inner ear.**
318   [17891714] Int J Dev Biol 51(6-7):521-33 (2007)

2007   **Shaping the mammalian auditory sensory organ by the planar cell polarity pathway.**
319   [17891715] Int J Dev Biol 51(6-7):535-47 (2007)

2007   **Axon guidance in the inner ear.**
320   [17891716] Int J Dev Biol 51(6-7):549-56 (2007)

2007   **A network of growth and transcription factors controls neuronal differentation and survival in the developing ear.**
321   [17891717] Int J Dev Biol 51(6-7):557-70 (2007)

2007   **Cellular commitment and differentiation in the organ of Corti.**
322   [17891718] Int J Dev Biol 51(6-7):571-83 (2007)

2007   **Development of the hair bundle and mechanotransduction.**
323   [17891720] Int J Dev Biol 51(6-7):597-608 (2007)

2007   **The molecular biology of ear development - "Twenty years are nothing".**
324   [17891706] Int J Dev Biol 51(6-7):429-38 (2007)

2007   **The preplacodal region: an ectodermal domain with multipotential progenitors that contribute to sense organs and cranial sensory ganglia.**
325   [17891708] Int J Dev Biol 51(6-7):447-61 (2007)

2007   **The first steps towards hearing: mechanisms of otic placode induction.**
326   [17891709] Int J Dev Biol 51(6-7):463-72 (2007)

2008   **Mouse induced pluripotent stem cells.**
327   [18956334] Int J Dev Biol 52(8):1015-22 (2008)

2008   **The Apical Ectodermal Ridge: morphological aspects and signaling pathways.**
328   [18956316] Int J Dev Biol 52(7):857-71 (2008)

2008   **Genes controlling pancreas ontogeny.**
329   [18956314] Int J Dev Biol 52(7):823-35 (2008)

2008   **Anuran and pig egg zona pellucida glycoproteins in fertilization and early development.**
330   [18649282] Int J Dev Biol 52(5-6):683-701 (2008)

2008   **Sperm head membrane reorganisation during capacitation.**
331   [18649260] Int J Dev Biol 52(5-6):473-80 (2008)

2008   **Puzzles of mammalian fertilization--and beyond.**
332   [18649254] Int J Dev Biol 52(5-6):415-26 (2008)

2008   **From planarians to mammals - the many faces of regeneration.**
333   [18311712] Int J Dev Biol 52(2-3):219-27 (2008)

2008   **On the transition from the meiotic to mitotic cell cycle during early mouse development.**
334   [18311711] Int J Dev Biol 52(2-3):201-17 (2008)

2010   **Electron cryotomography.**
335   [20516135] Cold Spring Harb Perspect Biol 2(6):a003442 (2010)

2010   **The Hadean-Archaean environment.**
336   [20516134] Cold Spring Harb Perspect Biol 2(6):a002527 (2010)

2010   **Guidance molecules in axon pruning and cell death.**
337   [20516131] Cold Spring Harb Perspect Biol 2(6):a001859 (2010)

2010   **Auxin control of root development.**
338   [20516130] Cold Spring Harb Perspect Biol 2(6):a001537 (2010)

2010   **The tumor suppressor p53: from structures to drug discovery.**
339   [20516128] Cold Spring Harb Perspect Biol 2(6):a000919 (2010)

2010   **Gene positioning.**
340   [20484389] Cold Spring Harb Perspect Biol 2(6):a000588 (2010)

2010   **Wiring the brain: the biology of neuronal guidance.**
341   [20463002] Cold Spring Harb Perspect Biol 2(6):a001917 (2010)

2011   **The growth cone cytoskeleton in axon outgrowth and guidance.**
342   [21106647] Cold Spring Harb Perspect Biol 3(3):- (2011)

2010   **RNA processing and export.**
343   [20961978] Cold Spring Harb Perspect Biol 2(12):a000752 (2010)

2010   **Chromosome territories.**
344   [20300217] Cold Spring Harb Perspect Biol 2(3):a003889 (2010)

2010   **The bacterial cell envelope.**
345   [20452953] Cold Spring Harb Perspect Biol 2(5):a000414 (2010)

2010   **Chromatin higher-order structure and dynamics.**
346   [20452954] Cold Spring Harb Perspect Biol 2(5):a000596 (2010)

2010   **Single-molecule and superresolution imaging in live bacteria cells.**
347   [20300204] Cold Spring Harb Perspect Biol 2(3):a000448 (2010)

2010   **The nuclear envelope.**
348   [20300205] Cold Spring Harb Perspect Biol 2(3):a000539 (2010)

2010   **Auxin and monocot development.**
349   [20300208] Cold Spring Harb Perspect Biol 2(3):a001479 (2010)

2010   **Auxin transporters--why so many?**
350   [20300209] Cold Spring Harb Perspect Biol 2(3):a001552 (2010)

2009
371
Vertebrate limb development: moving from classical morphogen gradients to an integrated 4-dimensional patterning system.
[20066096] Cold Spring Harb Perspect Biol 1(4):a001339 (2009)

2009
372
Control of NF-kappaB-dependent transcriptional responses by chromatin organization.
[20066094] Cold Spring Harb Perspect Biol 1(4):a000224 (2009)

2009
373
Discovering the molecular components of intercellular junctions--a historical view.
[20066111] Cold Spring Harb Perspect Biol 1(3):a003061 (2009)

2009
374
Structure and biochemistry of cadherins and catenins.
[20066110] Cold Spring Harb Perspect Biol 1(3):a003053 (2009)

2009
375
Planar cell polarity signaling: the developing cell's compass.
[20066108] Cold Spring Harb Perspect Biol 1(3):a002964 (2009)

2009
376
Modular design of immunological synapses and kinapses.
[20066081] Cold Spring Harb Perspect Biol 1(1):a002873 (2009)

2009
377
Gap junctions.
[20066080] Cold Spring Harb Perspect Biol 1(1):a002576 (2009)

2009
378
The measure of success: constraints, objectives, and tradeoffs in morphogen-mediated patterning.
[20066078] Cold Spring Harb Perspect Biol 1(1):a002022 (2009)

2009
379
Left-right determination: involvement of molecular motor KIF3, cilia, and nodal flow.
[20066075] Cold Spring Harb Perspect Biol 1(1):a000802 (2009)

2009
380
Remodeling epithelial cell organization: transitions between front-rear and apical-basal polarity.
[20066074] Cold Spring Harb Perspect Biol 1(1):a000513 (2009)

2010
381
The yin and yang of chromatin spatial organization.
[20353545] Genome Biol 11(3):204 (2010)

2009
382
Epigenetic transmission of piRNAs through the female germline.
[19232071] Genome Biol 10(2):208 (2009)

2007
383
Technology transfer from worms and flies to vertebrates: transposition-based genome manipulations and their future perspectives.
[18047686] Genome Biol 8 Suppl 1(-):S1 (2007)

2007
384
Decoding dosage compensation.
[17328790] Genome Biol 8(2):204 (2007)

2005
385
Histone modifications: from genome-wide maps to functional insights.
[15960810] Genome Biol 6(6):113 (2005)

2008
386
Linking genes to literature: text mining, information extraction, and retrieval applications for biology.
[18834499] Genome Biol 9 Suppl 2(-):S8 (2008)

2008
387
Mathematical models in mammalian cell biology.
[18638360] Genome Biol 9(7):316 (2008)

2008
388
The AID/APOBEC family of nucleic acid mutators.
[18598372] Genome Biol 9(6):229 (2008)

2008
389
Plant immunity from A to Z.
[18423060] Genome Biol 9(4):304 (2008)

2008   Bacterial pathogens encode suppressors of RNA-mediated silencing.
390   [18947381] Genome Biol 9(10):237 (2008)

2009   The netrin protein family.
391   [19785719] Genome Biol 10(9):239 (2009)

2009   Transposons that clean up after themselves.
392   [19589181] Genome Biol 10(6):224 (2009)

2006   Automatic annotation of eukaryotic genes, pseudogenes and promoters.
393   [16925832] Genome Biol 7 Suppl 1(-):S10.1-12 (2006)

2010   Systematic characterizations of text similarity in full text biomedical publications.
394   [20856807] PLoS One 5(9):e12704 (2010)

2010   Utilizing genotype imputation for the augmentation of sequence data.
395   [20543988] PLoS One 5(6):e11018 (2010)

2010   Insights in 17beta-HSD1 enzyme kinetics and ligand binding by dynamic motion investigation.
396   [20706575] PLoS One 5(8):e12026 (2010)

2011   Expression-based in silico screening of candidate therapeutic compounds for lung adenocarcinoma.
397   [21283735] PLoS One 6(1):e14573 (2011)

2011   Prediction of disease and phenotype associations from genome-wide association studies.
398   [22076134] PLoS One 6(11):e27175 (2011)

2011   Design considerations for massively parallel sequencing studies of complex human disease.
399   [21850262] PLoS One 6(8):e23221 (2011)

2011   On the lack of consensus over the meaning of openness: an empirical study.
400   [21858110] PLoS One 6(8):e23420 (2011)

2011   Using and reporting the Delphi method for selecting healthcare quality indicators: a systematic review.
401   [21694759] PLoS One 6(6):e20476 (2011)

2011   The development of open access journal publishing from 1993 to 2009.
402   [21695139] PLoS One 6(6):e20961 (2011)

2011   A meta-analysis of predation risk effects on pollinator behaviour.
403   [21695187] PLoS One 6(6):e20689 (2011)

2011   Choosing and using a plant DNA barcode.
404   [21637336] PLoS One 6(5):e19254 (2011)

2011   A propaganda index for reviewing problem framing in articles and manuscripts: an exploratory study.
405   [21647426] PLoS One 6(5):e19516 (2011)

2010   The promise and perils of pre-publication review: a multi-agent simulation of biomedical discovery under varying levels of review stringency.
406   [20520812] PLoS One 5(5):e10782 (2010)

2007   An outbreak of severe infections with community-acquired MRSA carrying the Panton-Valentine leukocidin following vaccination.
407   [17786194] PLoS One 2(9):e822 (2007)

2009   How many scientists fabricate and falsify research? A systematic review and meta-analysis of survey data.
408   [19478950] PLoS One 4(5):e5738 (2009)

2008
409
Toward a comprehensive approach to the collection and analysis of pica substances, with emphasis on geophagic materials.
[18773081] PLoS One 3(9):e3147 (2008)

2009
410
Discovery of the largest orbweaving spider species: the evolution of gigantism in Nephila.
[19844575] PLoS One 4(10):e7516 (2009)

2010
411
Neurophysiological and computational principles of cortical rhythms in cognition.
[20664082] Physiol Rev 90(3):1195-268 (2010)

2010
412
Fluorescent proteins and their applications in imaging living cells and tissues.
[20664080] Physiol Rev 90(3):1103-63 (2010)

2010
413
Mechanisms of sound localization in mammals.
[20664077] Physiol Rev 90(3):983-1012 (2010)

2010
414
Gut microbiota in health and disease.
[20664075] Physiol Rev 90(3):859-904 (2010)

2006
415
Thermogenic mechanisms and their hormonal regulation.
[16601266] Physiol Rev 86(2):435-64 (2006)

2002
416
The transporter associated with antigen processing: function and implications in human diseases.
[11773612] Physiol Rev 82(1):187-204 (2002)

2011
417
The WNKs: atypical protein kinases with pleiotropic actions.
[21248166] Physiol Rev 91(1):177-219 (2011)

2011
418
Hyaluronan as an immune regulator in human diseases.
[21248167] Physiol Rev 91(1):221-64 (2011)

2010
419
Fluid transport across leaky epithelia: central role of the tight junction and supporting role of aquaporins.
[20959616] Physiol Rev 90(4):1271-90 (2010)

2010
420
Mammalian Krüppel-like factors in health and diseases.
[20959618] Physiol Rev 90(4):1337-81 (2010)

2010
421
Regulation of mammalian autophagy in physiology and pathophysiology.
[20959619] Physiol Rev 90(4):1383-435 (2010)

2010
422
Ca2+-activated K+ channels: from protein complexes to function.
[20959620] Physiol Rev 90(4):1437-59 (2010)

2010
423
Proteases and proteolysis in Alzheimer disease: a multifactorial view on the disease process.
[20393191] Physiol Rev 90(2):465-94 (2010)

2010
424
Sympathetic nervous system overactivity and its role in the development of cardiovascular disease.
[20393193] Physiol Rev 90(2):513-57 (2010)

2010
425
Physiology of kidney renin.
[20393195] Physiol Rev 90(2):607-73 (2010)

2010
426
The ventilatory response to hypoxia in mammals: mechanisms, measurement, and analysis.
[20393196] Physiol Rev 90(2):675-754 (2010)

2010
427
Plastic synaptic networks of the amygdala for the acquisition, expression, and extinction of conditioned fear.
[20393190] Physiol Rev 90(2):419-63 (2010)

2005   **Hormonal regulation of food intake.**
428   [16183909] Physiol Rev 85(4):1131-58 (2005)

2004   **Mouse models of insulin resistance.**
429   [15044684] Physiol Rev 84(2):623-47 (2004)

2004   **Cellular and molecular regulation of muscle regeneration.**
430   [14715915] Physiol Rev 84(1):209-38 (2004)

2004   **Phosphoinositides in constitutive membrane traffic.**
431   [15269334] Physiol Rev 84(3):699-730 (2004)

2005   **Physiology and pathophysiology of the calcium store in the endoplasmic reticulum of neurons.**
432   [15618481] Physiol Rev 85(1):201-79 (2005)

2003   **Role of monocytes in atherogenesis.**
433   [14506301] Physiol Rev 83(4):1069-112 (2003)

2003   **Mammalian hibernation: cellular and molecular responses to depressed metabolism and low temperature.**
434   [14506303] Physiol Rev 83(4):1153-81 (2003)

2003   **Interaction of mycoplasmas with host cells.**
435   [12663864] Physiol Rev 83(2):417-32 (2003)

2003   **Regulation of amino acid and glucose transporters in endothelial and smooth muscle cells.**
436   [12506130] Physiol Rev 83(1):183-252 (2003)

2010   **The Fox genes in the liver: from organogenesis to functional integration.**
437   [20086072] Physiol Rev 90(1):1-22 (2010)

2010   **Pathophysiology of sleep apnea.**
438   [20086074] Physiol Rev 90(1):47-112 (2010)

2010   **Regulation of the actin cytoskeleton-plasma membrane interplay by phosphoinositides.**
439   [20086078] Physiol Rev 90(1):259-89 (2010)

2010   **Inwardly rectifying potassium channels: their structure, function, and physiological roles.**
440   [20086079] Physiol Rev 90(1):291-366 (2010)

2007   **GABA: a pioneer transmitter that excites immature neurons and generates primitive oscillations.**
441   [17928584] Physiol Rev 87(4):1215-84 (2007)

2007   **Transient receptor potential cation channels in disease.**
442   [17237345] Physiol Rev 87(1):165-217 (2007)

2009   **Mechanisms of cancer cachexia.**
443   [19342610] Physiol Rev 89(2):381-410 (2009)

2009   **Catecholaminergic systems in stress: structural and molecular genetic approaches.**
444   [19342614] Physiol Rev 89(2):535-606 (2009)

2009   **Alcoholism: a systems approach from molecular physiology to addictive behavior.**
445   [19342616] Physiol Rev 89(2):649-705 (2009)

2009   **Models and mechanisms of hyperalgesia and allodynia.**
446   [19342617] Physiol Rev 89(2):707-58 (2009)

2008   **Local gene expression in axons and nerve endings: the glia-neuron unit.**
447   [18391172] Physiol Rev 88(2):515-55 (2008)

2008   **Diffusion in brain extracellular space.**
448   [18923183] Physiol Rev 88(4):1277-340 (2008)

2005   **Controlling cell behavior electrically: current views and future potential.**
449   [15987799] Physiol Rev 85(3):943-78 (2005)

2009   **Muscle giants: molecular scaffolds in sarcomerogenesis.**
450   [19789381] Physiol Rev 89(4):1217-67 (2009)

2009   **Prions: protein aggregation and infectious diseases.**
451   [19789378] Physiol Rev 89(4):1105-52 (2009)

2009   **Aneuploidy: from a physiological mechanism of variance to Down syndrome.**
452   [19584316] Physiol Rev 89(3):887-920 (2009)

2009   **From pheromones to behavior.**
453   [19584317] Physiol Rev 89(3):921-56 (2009)

2009   **AMPK in Health and Disease.**
454   [19584320] Physiol Rev 89(3):1025-78 (2009)

2009   **Lung parenchymal mechanics in health and disease.**
455   [19584312] Physiol Rev 89(3):759-75 (2009)

2009   **LKB1 and AMPK family signaling: the intimate link between cell polarity and energy metabolism.**
456   [19584313] Physiol Rev 89(3):777-98 (2009)

2009   **Mitochondrial dynamics in mammalian health and disease.**
457   [19584314] Physiol Rev 89(3):799-845 (2009)

2010   **Autophagy, a guardian against neurodegeneration.**
458   [20188203] Semin Cell Dev Biol 21(7):691-8 (2010)

2010   **Chaperone-mediated autophagy: molecular mechanisms and physiological relevance.**
459   [20176123] Semin Cell Dev Biol 21(7):719-26 (2010)

2010   **Coordinating mitosis with cell polarity: Molecular motors at the cell cortex.**
460   [20109571] Semin Cell Dev Biol 21(3):283-9 (2010)

2007   **Lipid rafts, fluid/fluid phase separation, and their relevance to plasma membrane structure and function.**
461   [17764993] Semin Cell Dev Biol 18(5):583-90 (2007)

2007   **The role of insulator elements in large-scale chromatin structure in interphase.**
462   [17919949] Semin Cell Dev Biol 18(5):682-90 (2007)

2009   **Fluorescence microscopy below the diffraction limit.**
463   [19698798] Semin Cell Dev Biol 20(8):886-93 (2009)

2008   **Uterine receptivity to human embryonic implantation: histology, biomarkers, and transcriptomics.**
464   [18035563] Semin Cell Dev Biol 19(2):204-11 (2008)

2009   **Regulation of convergence and extension movements during vertebrate gastrulation by the Wnt/PCP pathway.**
465   [19761865] Semin Cell Dev Biol 20(8):986-97 (2009)

2010   **A guide to super-resolution fluorescence microscopy.**
466   [20643879] J Cell Biol 190(2):165-75 (2010)

2010   Review series: The cell biology of hearing.
467   [20624897] J Cell Biol 190(1):9-20 (2010)

2010   The cell biology of vision.
468   [20855501] J Cell Biol 190(6):953-63 (2010)

2010   Neighborly relations: cadherins and mechanotransduction.
469   [20584914] J Cell Biol 189(7):1075-7 (2010)

2010   Clearance of apoptotic cells: implications in health and disease.
470   [20584912] J Cell Biol 189(7):1059-70 (2010)

2010   Regulation of innate immune responses by autophagy-related proteins.
471   [20548099] J Cell Biol 189(6):925-35 (2010)

2010   The cell biology of taste.
472   [20696704] J Cell Biol 190(3):285-96 (2010)

2010   Mass spectrometry-based proteomics in cell biology.
473   [20733050] J Cell Biol 190(4):491-500 (2010)

2006   Drosophila Cajal bodies: accessories not included.
474   [16533940] J Cell Biol 172(6):791-3 (2006)

2006   RNA granules.
475   [16520386] J Cell Biol 172(6):803-8 (2006)

2011   Peroxisome assembly: matrix and membrane protein biogenesis.
476   [21464226] J Cell Biol 193(1):7-16 (2011)

2011   Four faces of cellular senescence.
477   [21321098] J Cell Biol 192(4):547-56 (2011)

2011   Circulating tumor cells: approaches to isolation and characterization.
478   [21300848] J Cell Biol 192(3):373-82 (2011)

2011   Dynamics of adherens junctions in epithelial establishment, maintenance, and remodeling.
479   [21422226] J Cell Biol 192(6):907-17 (2011)

2011   On emerging nuclear order.
480   [21383074] J Cell Biol 192(5):711-21 (2011)

2011   Principles of chromosomal organization: lessons from yeast.
481   [21383075] J Cell Biol 192(5):723-33 (2011)

2011   Lymphatic vascular morphogenesis in development, physiology, and disease.
482   [21576390] J Cell Biol 193(4):607-18 (2011)

2011   Regulating the transition from centriole to basal body.
483   [21536747] J Cell Biol 193(3):435-44 (2011)

2011   Mitochondrial DNA mutations in disease and aging.
484   [21606204] J Cell Biol 193(5):809-18 (2011)

2010   The cell biology of touch.
485   [20956378] J Cell Biol 191(2):237-48 (2010)

2010   The cell biology of smell.
486   [21041441] J Cell Biol 191(3):443-52 (2010)

2010	The cell biology of polycystic kidney disease.
487	[21079243] J Cell Biol 191(4):701-10 (2010)

2010	piRNAs, transposon silencing, and Drosophila germline development.
488	[21115802] J Cell Biol 191(5):905-13 (2010)

2010	Actin in dendritic spines: connecting dynamics to function.
489	[20457765] J Cell Biol 189(4):619-29 (2010)

2010	The immunological synapse: a focal point for endocytosis and exocytosis.
490	[20439993] J Cell Biol 189(3):399-406 (2010)

2010	Regulation of basal cellular physiology by the homeostatic unfolded protein response.
491	[20513765] J Cell Biol 189(5):783-94 (2010)

2010	Plasticity of cell migration: a multiscale tuning model.
492	[19951899] J Cell Biol 188(1):11-9 (2010)

2010	Pericentrin in cellular function and disease.
493	[19951897] J Cell Biol 188(2):181-90 (2010)

2010	Tapping into the glial reservoir: cells committed to remaining uncommitted.
494	[20142420] J Cell Biol 188(3):305-12 (2010)

2009	Assembly of multiprotein complexes that control genome function.
495	[19332890] J Cell Biol 185(1):21-6 (2009)

2007	Sending proteins to dense core secretory granules: still a lot to sort out.
496	[17438078] J Cell Biol 177(2):191-6 (2007)

2009	Bringing KASH under the SUN: the many faces of nucleo-cytoskeletal connections.
497	[19687252] J Cell Biol 186(4):461-72 (2009)

2008	The cell biological basis of ciliary disease.
498	[18180369] J Cell Biol 180(1):17-21 (2008)

2008	Intraflagellar transport motors in cilia: moving along the cell's antenna.
499	[18180368] J Cell Biol 180(1):23-9 (2008)

2008	Decoding ARE-mediated decay: is microRNA part of the equation?
500	[18411313] J Cell Biol 181(2):189-94 (2008)

2006	The chromosomal passenger complex: guiding Aurora-B through mitosis.
501	[16769825] J Cell Biol 173(6):833-7 (2006)

2010	The ZEB/miR-200 feedback loop--a motor of cellular plasticity in development and cancer?
502	[20706219] EMBO Rep 11(9):670-7 (2010)

2010	Mechanisms of force generation and force transmission during interstitial leukocyte migration.
503	[20865016] EMBO Rep 11(10):744-50 (2010)

2010	Further assembly required: construction and dynamics of the endoplasmic reticulum network.
504	[20559323] EMBO Rep 11(7):515-21 (2010)

2010	The history of p53. A perfect example of the drawbacks of scientific paradigms.
505	[20930848] EMBO Rep 11(11):822-6 (2010)

2004	A topological view of the replicon.
506	[14993926] EMBO Rep 5(3):256-61 (2004)

2005
507

RNA sequence- and shape-dependent recognition by proteins in the ribonucleoprotein particle.
[15643449] EMBO Rep 6(1):33-8 (2005)

2003
508

Ring, helix, sphere and cylinder: the basic geometry of prokaryotic cell division.
[12835751] EMBO Rep 4(7):655-60 (2003)

2007
509

Like father like son. A fresh review of the inheritance of acquired characteristics.
[17767188] EMBO Rep 8(9):798-803 (2007)

2007
510

A variable topology for the 30-nm chromatin fibre.
[18059311] EMBO Rep 8(12):1129-34 (2007)

2009
511

Linear polyubiquitination: a new regulator of NF-kappaB activation.
[19543231] EMBO Rep 10(7):706-13 (2009)

2005
512

Letter from the editor: Adenosine-to-inosine RNA editing in Alu repeats in the human genome.
[16138094] EMBO Rep 6(9):831-5 (2005)

2005
513

DNA polymerases and somatic hypermutation of immunoglobulin genes.
[16319960] EMBO Rep 6(12):1143-8 (2005)

2008
514

The expanding field of poly(ADP-ribosyl)ation reactions. 'Protein Modifications: Beyond the Usual Suspects' Review Series.
[18927583] EMBO Rep 9(11):1094-100 (2008)

2006
515

Viroids: an Ariadne's thread into the RNA labyrinth.
[16741503] EMBO Rep 7(6):593-8 (2006)

2008
516

Grab, stick, pull and digest: the functional diversity of actin-associated matrix-adhesion structures. Workshop on Invadopodia, Podosomes and Focal Adhesions in Tissue Invasion.
[18202718] EMBO Rep 9(2):139-43 (2008)

2006
517

The science and ethics of making part-human animals in stem cell biology.
[16675841] FASEB J 20(7):838-45 (2006)

2010
518

Does oxidative stress contribute to the pathology of Friedreich's ataxia? A radical question.
[20219987] FASEB J 24(7):2152-63 (2010)

2010
519

Beta arcades: recurring motifs in naturally occurring and disease-related amyloid fibrils.
[20032312] FASEB J 24(5):1311-9 (2010)

2010
520

A generalized model of gene dosage and dominant negative effects in macromolecular complexes.
[20007508] FASEB J 24(4):994-1002 (2010)

2009
521

Epigenetics: poly(ADP-ribosyl)ation of PARP-1 regulates genomic methylation patterns.
[19001527] FASEB J 23(3):672-8 (2009)

2010
522

Generic binding sites, generic DNA-binding domains: where does specific promoter recognition come from?
[19762556] FASEB J 24(2):346-56 (2010)

2010
523

The P2X7 purinergic receptor: from physiology to neurological disorders.
[19812374] FASEB J 24(2):337-45 (2010)

2010
524

Lymphangiogenesis: in vitro and in vivo models.
[19726757] FASEB J 24(1):8-21 (2010)

2009
525

Structural insights on physiological functions and pathological effects of alpha-synuclein.
[18948383] FASEB J 23(2):329-40 (2009)

2007 **Human skin pigmentation: melanocytes modulate skin color in response to stress.**
526 [17242160] FASEB J 21(4):976-94 (2007)

2007 **Resolution of inflammation: state of the art, definitions and terms.**
527 [17267386] FASEB J 21(2):325-32 (2007)

2005 **Nanomedicine: current status and future prospects.**
528 [15746175] FASEB J 19(3):311-30 (2005)

2009 **SIRT1 controls circadian clock circuitry and promotes cell survival: a connection with age-related neoplasms.**
529 [19439501] FASEB J 23(9):2803-9 (2009)

2009 **Glucocorticoid-induced leucine zipper (GILZ): a new important mediator of glucocorticoid action.**
530 [19567371] FASEB J 23(11):3649-58 (2009)

2008 **Molecular and cellular aspects of protein misfolding and disease.**
531 [18303094] FASEB J 22(7):2115-33 (2008)

2008 **ADAM-15: a metalloprotease that mediates inflammation.**
532 [17905725] FASEB J 22(3):641-53 (2008)

2008 **The unexpected role of acid sphingomyelinase in cell death and the pathophysiology of common diseases.**
533 [18567738] FASEB J 22(10):3419-31 (2008)

2010 **The family of ubiquitin-conjugating enzymes (E2s): deciding between life and death of proteins.**
534 [19940261] FASEB J 24(4):981-93 (2010)

2009 **The mechanism of ABC transporters: general lessons from structural and functional studies of an antigenic peptide transporter.**
535 [19174475] FASEB J 23(5):1287-302 (2009)

2006 **A brief history of RNAi: the silence of the genes.**
536 [16816104] FASEB J 20(9):1293-9 (2006)

2002 **Blood coagulation.**
537 [11841335] Biochemistry (Mosc) 67(1):3-12 (2002)

2002 **Contact system. New concepts on activation mechanisms and bioregulatory functions.**
538 [11841336] Biochemistry (Mosc) 67(1):13-24 (2002)

2002 **Genetic mechanisms of hereditary hemostasis disorders.**
539 [11841338] Biochemistry (Mosc) 67(1):33-46 (2002)

2002 **The blood platelet as a model for regulating blood coagulation on cell surfaces and its consequences.**
540 [11841339] Biochemistry (Mosc) 67(1):47-55 (2002)

2002 **Thrombin regulation of cell function through protease-activated receptors: implications for therapeutic intervention.**
541 [11841340] Biochemistry (Mosc) 67(1):56-64 (2002)

2002 **Receptors of the PAR family as a link between blood coagulation and inflammation.**
542 [11841341] Biochemistry (Mosc) 67(1):65-74 (2002)

2002 **Molecular mechanisms of thrombin-induced endothelial cell permeability.**
543 [11841342] Biochemistry (Mosc) 67(1):75-84 (2002)

2002 **Matrix metalloproteinases and cellular fibrinolytic activity.**
544 [11841344] Biochemistry (Mosc) 67(1):92-8 (2002)

2002   **The fibrinolysis system: regulation of activity and physiologic functions of its main components.**
545   [11841345] Biochemistry (Mosc) 67(1):99-108 (2002)

2008   **Mechanisms of angiogenesis.**
546   [18707583] Biochemistry (Mosc) 73(7):751-62 (2008)

2004   **Short forms of membrane receptors: generation and role in hormonal signal transduction.**
547   [15170369] Biochemistry (Mosc) 69(4):351-63 (2004)

2004   **Properties, functions, and secretion of human myeloperoxidase.**
548   [14972011] Biochemistry (Mosc) 69(1):4-9 (2004)

2004   **Photobiological principles of therapeutic applications of laser radiation.**
549   [14972023] Biochemistry (Mosc) 69(1):81-90 (2004)

2004   **Molecular architecture of bacteriophage T4.**
550   [15627372] Biochemistry (Mosc) 69(11):1190-202 (2004)

2004   **Electron tomography of biological samples.**
551   [15627375] Biochemistry (Mosc) 69(11):1219-25 (2004)

2004   **Biochemical problems of regulation by oligopeptides.**
552   [15627381] Biochemistry (Mosc) 69(11):1276-82 (2004)

2005   **Persister cells and the riddle of biofilm survival.**
553   [15807669] Biochemistry (Mosc) 70(2):267-74 (2005)

2005   **Role of cooperative H(+)/e(-) linkage (redox bohr effect) at heme a/Cu(A) and heme a(3)/Cu(B) in the proton pump of cytochrome c oxidase.**
554   [15807657] Biochemistry (Mosc) 70(2):178-86 (2005)

2005   **A historical review of cellular calcium handling, with emphasis on mitochondria.**
555   [15807658] Biochemistry (Mosc) 70(2):187-94 (2005)

2005   **Lipophilic triphenylphosphonium cations as tools in mitochondrial bioenergetics and free radical biology.**
556   [15807662] Biochemistry (Mosc) 70(2):222-30 (2005)

2005   **Programmed cell death via mitochondria: different modes of dying.**
557   [15807663] Biochemistry (Mosc) 70(2):231-9 (2005)

2005   **Proton transfer dynamics at membrane/water interface and mechanism of biological energy conversion.**
558   [15807666] Biochemistry (Mosc) 70(2):251-6 (2005)

2005   **Dielectric and photoelectric properties of photosynthetic reaction centers.**
559   [15807667] Biochemistry (Mosc) 70(2):257-63 (2005)

2005   **Cardiolipin in energy transducing membranes.**
560   [15807653] Biochemistry (Mosc) 70(2):154-8 (2005)

2005   **Involvement of mitochondrial inner membrane anion carriers in the uncoupling effect of fatty acids.**
561   [15807654] Biochemistry (Mosc) 70(2):159-63 (2005)

2009   **Proteasome system of protein degradation and processing.**
562   [20210701] Biochemistry (Mosc) 74(13):1411-42 (2009)

2009   **Principles of control over formation of structures responsible for respiratory functions of mitochondria.**
563   [20210702] Biochemistry (Mosc) 74(13):1443-56 (2009)

2009   **Nicking endonucleases.**
564   [20210703] Biochemistry (Mosc) 74(13):1457-66 (2009)

2009   **Structure and mechanism of action of type IA DNA topoisomerases.**
565   [20210704] Biochemistry (Mosc) 74(13):1467-81 (2009)

2009   **From structure and functions of steroidogenic enzymes to new technologies of gene engineering.**
566   [20210705] Biochemistry (Mosc) 74(13):1482-504 (2009)

2009   **Molecular diversity of spider venom.**
567   [20210706] Biochemistry (Mosc) 74(13):1505-34 (2009)

2009   **Free radicals and cell chemiluminescence.**
568   [20210708] Biochemistry (Mosc) 74(13):1545-66 (2009)

2009   **Modular nanotransporters of anticancer drugs conferring cell specificity and higher efficiency.**
569   [20210709] Biochemistry (Mosc) 74(13):1567-74 (2009)

2009   **Dynamic proteomics in modeling of the living cell. Protein-protein interactions.**
570   [20210711] Biochemistry (Mosc) 74(13):1586-607 (2009)

2007   **A comparison of catalytic site intermediates of cytochrome c oxidase and peroxidases.**
571   [18021063] Biochemistry (Mosc) 72(10):1047-55 (2007)

2007   **Primary mechanisms of photoactivation of molecular oxygen. History of development and the modern status of research.**
572   [18021065] Biochemistry (Mosc) 72(10):1065-80 (2007)

2007   **Mechanisms of oxidative modification of low density lipoproteins under conditions of oxidative and carbonyl stress.**
573   [18021066] Biochemistry (Mosc) 72(10):1081-90 (2007)

2007   **Nucleocytoplasmic transport of proteins.**
574   [18282135] Biochemistry (Mosc) 72(13):1439-57 (2007)

2007   **Effect of molecular crowding on the enzymes of glycogenolysis.**
575   [18282137] Biochemistry (Mosc) 72(13):1478-90 (2007)

2007   **Biological activity of hemoprotein nitrosyl complexes.**
576   [18282138] Biochemistry (Mosc) 72(13):1491-504 (2007)

2007   **Methods for selection of aptamers to protein targets.**
577   [18282139] Biochemistry (Mosc) 72(13):1505-18 (2007)

2007   **Prions.**
578   [18282140] Biochemistry (Mosc) 72(13):1519-36 (2007)

2007   **Versatile functions of p53 protein in multicellular organisms.**
579   [18282133] Biochemistry (Mosc) 72(13):1399-421 (2007)

2007   **Noncoding RNAs and chromatin structure.**
580   [18282134] Biochemistry (Mosc) 72(13):1422-38 (2007)

2008   **Nanocolonies: detection, cloning, and analysis of individual molecules.**
581   [19216706] Biochemistry (Mosc) 73(13):1361-87 (2008)

2008   **Mechanisms of single-stranded DNA-binding protein functioning in cellular DNA metabolism.**
582   [19216707] Biochemistry (Mosc) 73(13):1388-404 (2008)

2008 **Specific features of 5S rRNA structure - its interactions with macromolecules and possible functions.**
583   [19216709] Biochemistry (Mosc) 73(13):1418-37 (2008)

2008 **Embryonic stem cells and the problem of directed differentiation.**
584   [19216710] Biochemistry (Mosc) 73(13):1438-52 (2008)

2008 **Intermediate vimentin filaments and their role in intracellular organelle distribution.**
585   [19216711] Biochemistry (Mosc) 73(13):1453-66 (2008)

2008 **Capping complex formation at the slow-growing end of the actin filament.**
586   [19216712] Biochemistry (Mosc) 73(13):1467-72 (2008)

2008 **Involvement of thio-, peroxi-, and glutaredoxins in cellular redox-dependent processes.**
587   [19216714] Biochemistry (Mosc) 73(13):1493-510 (2008)

2008 **The problem of the eukaryotic genome size.**
588   [19216716] Biochemistry (Mosc) 73(13):1519-52 (2008)

2005 **Enzymatic DNA methylation is an epigenetic control for genetic functions of the cell.**
589   [15948703] Biochemistry (Mosc) 70(5):488-99 (2005)

2005 **DNA methylation and epigenotypes.**
590   [15948704] Biochemistry (Mosc) 70(5):500-4 (2005)

2005 **On the biological significance of DNA methylation.**
591   [15948705] Biochemistry (Mosc) 70(5):505-24 (2005)

2005 **Methylation of DNA--one of the major epigenetic markers.**
592   [15948706] Biochemistry (Mosc) 70(5):525-32 (2005)

2005 **DNA methylation and demethylation as targets for anticancer therapy.**
593   [15948707] Biochemistry (Mosc) 70(5):533-49 (2005)

2005 **The language of methylation in genomics of eukaryotes.**
594   [15948712] Biochemistry (Mosc) 70(5):584-95 (2005)

2008 **Transport proteins of the ABC family and multidrug resistance of tumor cells.**
595   [18605983] Biochemistry (Mosc) 73(5):592-604 (2008)

2008 **Tissue-specific transcription factors in progression of epithelial tumors.**
596   [18605982] Biochemistry (Mosc) 73(5):573-91 (2008)

2008 **Cancer-associated antigens and antigen arrays in serological diagnostics of malignant tumors.**
597   [18605981] Biochemistry (Mosc) 73(5):562-72 (2008)

2008 **Reorganization of molecular morphology of epitheliocytes and connective-tissue cells in**
598   **morphogenesis and carcinogenesis.**
       [18605977] Biochemistry (Mosc) 73(5):528-31 (2008)

2008 **On the path to understanding the nature of cancer.**
599   [18605973] Biochemistry (Mosc) 73(5):487-97 (2008)

2010 **Tumor necrosis factor-alpha converting enzyme: Implications for ocular inflammatory diseases.**
600   [20303413] Int J Biochem Cell Biol 42(7):1076-9 (2010)

2010 **The glomerulus--a view from the outside--the podocyte.**
601   [20542138] Int J Biochem Cell Biol 42(9):1380-7 (2010)

2010 **Cellular functions of transient receptor potential channels.**
602   [20399884] Int J Biochem Cell Biol 42(9):1430-45 (2010)

2010
603
Paramyxovirus assembly and budding: building particles that transmit infections.
[20398786] Int J Biochem Cell Biol 42(9):1416-29 (2010)

2010
604
Nlrp3: an immune sensor of cellular stress and infection.
[20079456] Int J Biochem Cell Biol 42(6):792-5 (2010)

2010
605
Nlrc4/Ipaf/CLAN/CARD12: more than a flagellin sensor.
[20067841] Int J Biochem Cell Biol 42(6):789-91 (2010)

2010
606
Lipolysis in adipocytes.
[20025992] Int J Biochem Cell Biol 42(5):555-9 (2010)

2004
607
The thrombospondins.
[15094109] Int J Biochem Cell Biol 36(6):961-8 (2004)

2010
608
Aldose reductase: a novel therapeutic target for inflammatory pathologies.
[19778627] Int J Biochem Cell Biol 42(1):17-20 (2010)

2009
609
O-GlcNAc cycling: implications for neurodegenerative disorders.
[19782947] Int J Biochem Cell Biol 41(11):2134-46 (2009)

2009
610
From mitochondrial dynamics to arrhythmias.
[19703656] Int J Biochem Cell Biol 41(10):1940-8 (2009)

2009
611
The role of PTEN-induced kinase 1 in mitochondrial dysfunction and dynamics.
[19703660] Int J Biochem Cell Biol 41(10):2025-35 (2009)

2009
612
Reversal of HIV-1 latency with anti-microRNA inhibitors.
[18761423] Int J Biochem Cell Biol 41(3):451-4 (2009)

2007
613
CD36: implications in cardiovascular disease.
[17466567] Int J Biochem Cell Biol 39(11):2012-30 (2007)

2007
614
Vascular endothelial growth factor: biology and therapeutic applications.
[17537667] Int J Biochem Cell Biol 39(7-8):1349-57 (2007)

2007
615
Control of cell fate and differentiation by Sry-related high-mobility-group box (Sox) transcription factors.
[17625949] Int J Biochem Cell Biol 39(12):2195-214 (2007)

2009
616
Potential therapeutic effects of curcumin, the anti-inflammatory agent, against neurodegenerative, cardiovascular, pulmonary, metabolic, autoimmune and neoplastic diseases.
[18662800] Int J Biochem Cell Biol 41(1):40-59 (2009)

2009
617
HIC1 (Hypermethylated in Cancer 1) epigenetic silencing in tumors.
[18723112] Int J Biochem Cell Biol 41(1):26-33 (2009)

2009
618
Phosphatase and tensin homologue deleted on chromosome 10: extending its PTENtacles.
[18950730] Int J Biochem Cell Biol 41(4):757-61 (2009)

2009
619
Multi-scale mechanics from molecules to morphogenesis.
[19394436] Int J Biochem Cell Biol 41(11):2147-62 (2009)

2009
620
Structural and functional link between the mitochondrial network and the endoplasmic reticulum.
[19389485] Int J Biochem Cell Biol 41(10):1817-27 (2009)

2009
621
Functions and mechanisms of action of CCN matricellular proteins.
[18775791] Int J Biochem Cell Biol 41(4):771-83 (2009)

2009
622
Regenerative pharmacology in the treatment of genetic diseases: the paradigm of muscular dystrophy.
[18804548] Int J Biochem Cell Biol 41(4):701-10 (2009)

2008
623
Extracellular calcium as an integrator of tissue function.
[18328773] Int J Biochem Cell Biol 40(8):1467-80 (2008)

2008
624
Fragments of extracellular matrix as mediators of inflammation.
[18243041] Int J Biochem Cell Biol 40(6-7):1101-10 (2008)

2008
625
The function of the NADPH oxidase of phagocytes and its relationship to other NOXs in plants, invertebrates, and mammals.
[18036868] Int J Biochem Cell Biol 40(4):604-18 (2008)

2008
626
Bridging structure with function: structural, regulatory, and developmental role of laminins.
[17855154] Int J Biochem Cell Biol 40(2):199-214 (2008)

2010
627
Fibrocytes: bringing new insights into mechanisms of inflammation and fibrosis.
[19850147] Int J Biochem Cell Biol 42(4):535-42 (2010)

2011
628
Role of Wnt/$\hat{I}^2$-catenin signaling in liver metabolism and cancer.
[19747566] Int J Biochem Cell Biol 43(7):1021-9 (2011)

2010
629
Choreographing an enzyme's dance.
[20822946] Curr Opin Chem Biol 14(5):636-43 (2010)

2010
630
Privileged scaffolds for library design and drug discovery.
[20303320] Curr Opin Chem Biol 14(3):347-61 (2010)

2010
631
Expanding the range of 'druggable' targets with natural product-based libraries: an academic perspective.
[20202892] Curr Opin Chem Biol 14(3):308-14 (2010)

2010
632
Fluorescent protein-based biosensors: resolving spatiotemporal dynamics of signaling.
[19910237] Curr Opin Chem Biol 14(1):37-42 (2010)

2010
633
Mitochondrial-targeted fluorescent probes for reactive oxygen species.
[19910238] Curr Opin Chem Biol 14(1):50-6 (2010)

2010
634
NIR dyes for bioimaging applications.
[19926332] Curr Opin Chem Biol 14(1):64-70 (2010)

2010
635
Visualizing protein-DNA interactions at the single-molecule level.
[19945909] Curr Opin Chem Biol 14(1):15-22 (2010)

2007
636
Argonautes confront new small RNAs.
[17928262] Curr Opin Chem Biol 11(5):569-77 (2007)

2007
637
Model systems for understanding DNA base pairing.
[17967435] Curr Opin Chem Biol 11(6):588-94 (2007)

2007
638
Model membrane systems and their applications.
[17976391] Curr Opin Chem Biol 11(6):581-7 (2007)

2007
639
RNA catalysis: ribozymes, ribosomes, and riboswitches.
[17981494] Curr Opin Chem Biol 11(6):636-43 (2007)

2008
640
Contemporary strategies for the stabilization of peptides in the alpha-helical conformation.
[18793750] Curr Opin Chem Biol 12(6):692-7 (2008)

2008
641

A repulsive field: advances in the electrostatics of the ion atmosphere.
[19081286] Curr Opin Chem Biol 12(6):619-25 (2008)

2009
642

Uncovering novel biochemistry in the mechanism of tryptophan tryptophylquinone cofactor biosynthesis.
[19648051] Curr Opin Chem Biol 13(4):469-74 (2009)

2008
643

Cofactor biosynthesis--still yielding fascinating new biological chemistry.
[18314013] Curr Opin Chem Biol 12(2):118-25 (2008)

2008
644

Nanowire sensors for multiplexed detection of biomolecules.
[18804551] Curr Opin Chem Biol 12(5):522-8 (2008)

2009
645

Hexosamine analogs: from metabolic glycoengineering to drug discovery.
[19747874] Curr Opin Chem Biol 13(5-6):565-72 (2009)

2009
646

Pyridoxal 5'-phosphate: electrophilic catalyst extraordinaire.
[19640775] Curr Opin Chem Biol 13(4):475-83 (2009)

2008
647

Discovering mechanisms of signaling-mediated cysteine oxidation.
[18282483] Curr Opin Chem Biol 12(1):18-24 (2008)

2006
648

Autophagy signaling and the cogwheels of cancer.
[16874041] Autophagy 2(2):67-73 (2006)

2011
649

Regulation of autophagy by lysosomal positioning.
[21521941] Autophagy 7(8):927-8 (2011)

2011
650

Selective autophagy mediated by autophagic adapter proteins.
[21189453] Autophagy 7(3):279-96 (2011)

2010
651

Assessing autophagy in the context of photodynamic therapy.
[19855190] Autophagy 6(1):7-18 (2010)

2010
652

Larval midgut destruction in Drosophila: not dependent on caspases but suppressed by the loss of autophagy.
[20009534] Autophagy 6(1):163-5 (2010)

2010
653

Autophagy and adipogenesis: implications in obesity and type II diabetes.
[20110772] Autophagy 6(1):179-81 (2010)

2006
654

Deficiency in apoptotic effectors Bax and Bak reveals an autophagic cell death pathway initiated by photodamage to the endoplasmic reticulum.
[16874066] Autophagy 2(3):238-40 (2006)

2010
655

Transitions between epithelial and mesenchymal states and the morphogenesis of the early mouse embryo.
[20200481] Cell Adh Migr 4(3):447-57 (2010)

2011
656

Filopodia initiation: focus on the Arp2/3 complex and formins.
[21975549] Cell Adh Migr 5(5):402-8 (2011)

2011
657

Filopodia and adhesion in cancer cell motility.
[21975551] Cell Adh Migr 5(5):421-30 (2011)

2011
658

Epithelial delamination and migration: lessons from Drosophila.
[21836393] Cell Adh Migr 5(4):366-72 (2011)

2010
659

Control of neural crest cell behavior and migration: Insights from live imaging.
[20671421] Cell Adh Migr 4(4):586-94 (2010)

2010   **Snail: More than EMT.**
660   [20168078] Cell Adh Migr 4(2):199-203 (2010)

2010   **New therapeutic strategies targeting transmembrane signal transduction in the immune system.**
661   [20519929] Cell Adh Migr 4(2):255-67 (2010)

2010   **Guidance molecules in lung cancer.**
662   [20139699] Cell Adh Migr 4(1):130-45 (2010)

2010   **Roles of E3 ubiquitin ligases in cell adhesion and migration.**
663   [20009572] Cell Adh Migr 4(1):10-8 (2010)

2007   **Amoeboid chemotaxis: future challenges and opportunities.**
664   [19262145] Cell Adh Migr 1(4):165-70 (2007)

2007   **From tango to quadrilla: current views of the immunological synapse.**
665   [19262090] Cell Adh Migr 1(1):7-12 (2007)

2007   **Viewing malignant melanoma cells as macrophage-tumor hybrids.**
666   [19262091] Cell Adh Migr 1(1):2-6 (2007)

2009   **Neurovascular development: The beginning of a beautiful friendship.**
667   [19363295] Cell Adh Migr 3(2):199-204 (2009)

2009   **Integrin-mediated regulation of neurovascular development, physiology and disease.**
668   [19372738] Cell Adh Migr 3(2):211-5 (2009)

2009   **An amicable separation: Chick's way of doing EMT.**
669   [19262172] Cell Adh Migr 3(2):160-3 (2009)

2009   **PtdIns(3,4)P2 instigates focal adhesions to generate podosomes.**
670   [19262173] Cell Adh Migr 3(2):195-7 (2009)

2009   **Cell lineages and early patterns of embryonic CNS vascularization.**
671   [19270493] Cell Adh Migr 3(2):205-10 (2009)

2009   **Advances and perspectives of the architecture of hemidesmosomes: lessons from structural biology.**
672   [19736524] Cell Adh Migr 3(4):361-4 (2009)

2009   **Multiple signaling interactions coordinate collective cell migration of the posterior lateral line primordium.**
673   [19736513] Cell Adh Migr 3(4):365-8 (2009)

2009   **Quantitative real-time imaging of molecular dynamics during cancer cell invasion and metastasis in vivo.**
674   [19690469] Cell Adh Migr 3(4):351-4 (2009)

2009   **The coordination between actin filaments and adhesion in mesenchymal migration.**
675   [19684475] Cell Adh Migr 3(4):355-7 (2009)

2009   **Anchoring stem cells in the niche by cell adhesion molecules.**
676   [19421010] Cell Adh Migr 3(4):396-401 (2009)

2009   **The role of the transcriptional regulator snail in cell detachment, reattachment and migration.**
677   [19287205] Cell Adh Migr 3(3):259-63 (2009)

2009   **SRF in angiogenesis: branching the vascular system.**
678   [19287204] Cell Adh Migr 3(3):264-7 (2009)

2010   **Cellular dynamics in the early mouse embryo: from axis formation to gastrulation.**
679   [20566281] Curr Opin Genet Dev 20(4):420-7 (2010)

2010   **RNAi-dependent formation of heterochromatin and its diverse functions.**
680   [20207534] Curr Opin Genet Dev 20(2):134-41 (2010)

2010   **RNA traffic control of chromatin complexes.**
681   [20362426] Curr Opin Genet Dev 20(2):142-8 (2010)

2008   **Back and forth between cell fate specification and movement during vertebrate gastrulation.**
682   [18721878] Curr Opin Genet Dev 18(4):311-6 (2008)

2008   **Message in a nucleus: signaling to the transcriptional machinery.**
683   [18678250] Curr Opin Genet Dev 18(5):397-403 (2008)

2005   **Tumor-stroma interactions.**
684   [15661539] Curr Opin Genet Dev 15(1):97-101 (2005)

2010   **The ups and downs of Myc biology.**
685   [19962879] Curr Opin Genet Dev 20(1):91-5 (2010)

2010   **HIF-1: upstream and downstream of cancer metabolism.**
686   [19942427] Curr Opin Genet Dev 20(1):51-6 (2010)

2010   **Intravital imaging of stromal cell dynamics in tumors.**
687   [19942428] Curr Opin Genet Dev 20(1):72-8 (2010)

2010   **Paramutation in maize: RNA mediated trans-generational gene silencing.**
688   [20153628] Curr Opin Genet Dev 20(2):156-63 (2010)

2007   **We gather together: insulators and genome organization.**
689   [17913488] Curr Opin Genet Dev 17(5):400-7 (2007)

2009   **Emerging pathogenic pathways in the spinocerebellar ataxias.**
690   [19345087] Curr Opin Genet Dev 19(3):247-53 (2009)

2009   **Lipid-modified morphogens: functions of fats.**
691   [19442512] Curr Opin Genet Dev 19(4):308-14 (2009)

2009   **The RASopathies: developmental syndromes of Ras/MAPK pathway dysregulation.**
692   [19467855] Curr Opin Genet Dev 19(3):230-6 (2009)

2009   **The primary cilium as a cellular signaling center: lessons from disease.**
693   [19477114] Curr Opin Genet Dev 19(3):220-9 (2009)

2009   **Duplication hotspots, rare genomic disorders, and common disease.**
694   [19477115] Curr Opin Genet Dev 19(3):196-204 (2009)

2008   **siRNA and miRNA processing: new functions for Cajal bodies.**
695   [18337083] Curr Opin Genet Dev 18(2):197-203 (2008)

2009   **Kidney development: from ureteric bud formation to branching morphogenesis.**
696   [19828308] Curr Opin Genet Dev 19(5):484-90 (2009)

2009   **Bringing together components of the fly renal system.**
697   [19783135] Curr Opin Genet Dev 19(5):526-32 (2009)

2008   **The transition from transcriptional initiation to elongation.**
698   [18282700] Curr Opin Genet Dev 18(2):130-6 (2008)

2006
699
Cellular and molecular mechanisms of synovial joint and articular cartilage formation.
[16831907] Ann N Y Acad Sci 1068(-):74-86 (2006)

2010
700
Bioenergetics and cell death.
[20649539] Ann N Y Acad Sci 1201(-):50-7 (2010)

2010
701
REM sleep behavior disorder: Updated review of the core features, the REM sleep behavior disorder-neurodegenerative disease association, evolving concepts, controversies, and future directions.
[20146689] Ann N Y Acad Sci 1184(-):15-54 (2010)

2010
702
Development of thymically derived natural regulatory T cells.
[20146704] Ann N Y Acad Sci 1183(-):1-12 (2010)

2010
703
Thymic stromal lymphopoietin.
[20146705] Ann N Y Acad Sci 1183(-):13-24 (2010)

2010
704
A role for calreticulin in the pathogenesis of rheumatoid arthritis.
[20958321] Ann N Y Acad Sci 1209(-):91-8 (2010)

2010
705
Mechanisms of chylomicron uptake into lacteals.
[20961306] Ann N Y Acad Sci 1207 Suppl 1(-):E52-7 (2010)

2008
706
Enzymology of the wood-Ljungdahl pathway of acetogenesis.
[18378591] Ann N Y Acad Sci 1125(-):129-36 (2008)

2006
707
The emerging functionality of endogenous lectins: A primer to the concept and a case study on galectins including medical implications.
[16642727] Chang Gung Med J 29(1):37-62 (2006)

2006
708
Embryo-endometrial interaction.
[16642724] Chang Gung Med J 29(1):9-14 (2006)

2006
709
Management of posttraumatic enophthalmos.
[16924886] Chang Gung Med J 29(3):251-61 (2006)

2011
710
Direct activation of Bmi1 by Twist1: implications in cancer stemness, epithelial-mesenchymal transition, and clinical significance.
[21733352] Chang Gung Med J 34(3):229-38 (2011)

2010
711
Orbital blow-out fractures in children: characterization and surgical outcome.
[20584509] Chang Gung Med J 33(3):313-20 (2010)

2005
712
Brugada syndrome--an update.
[15880981] Chang Gung Med J 28(2):69-76 (2005)

2010
713
Heme oxygenase-1 in cardiovascular diseases: molecular mechanisms and clinical perspectives.
[20184791] Chang Gung Med J 33(1):13-24 (2010)

2010
714
Neonatal vitamin-responsive epileptic encephalopathies.
[20184790] Chang Gung Med J 33(1):1-12 (2010)

2007
715
New insights into the role of the ubiquitin-proteasome pathway in the regulation of apoptosis.
[18350730] Chang Gung Med J 30(6):469-79 (2007)

2007
716
The role of proximal tubular cells in interstitial fibrosis: understanding TGF-beta1.
[17477023] Chang Gung Med J 30(1):2-6 (2007)

2007
717
Leptospirosis in Taiwan--an underestimated infectious disease.
[17595998] Chang Gung Med J 30(2):109-15 (2007)

2007
718
Carbohydrate antigen sialyl Lewis a--its pathophysiological significance and induction mechanism in cancer progression.
[17760270] Chang Gung Med J 30(3):189-209 (2007)

2009
719
The potential application of granulocyte colony stimulating factor therapy on neuropathic pain.
[19527602] Chang Gung Med J 32(3):235-46 (2009)

2005
720
The cytokine activity of HMGB1--extracellular escape of the nuclear protein.
[16382751] Chang Gung Med J 28(10):673-82 (2005)

2008
721
Overview of laser refractive surgery.
[18782946] Chang Gung Med J 31(3):237-52 (2008)

2008
722
Analysis of protein phosphorylation using mass spectrometry.
[18782944] Chang Gung Med J 31(3):217-27 (2008)

2005
723
Diagnostic approach to recurrent bacterial meningitis in children.
[16231527] Chang Gung Med J 28(7):441-52 (2005)

2008
724
Immune intervention with monoclonal antibodies targeting CD152 (CTLA-4) for autoimmune and malignant diseases.
[18419049] Chang Gung Med J 31(1):1-15 (2008)

2006
725
Mammalian nuclear transfer.
[16881069] Dev Dyn 235(9):2460-9 (2006)

2010
726
How does the tubular embryonic heart work? Looking for the physical mechanism generating unidirectional blood flow in the valveless embryonic heart tube.
[20235196] Dev Dyn 239(4):1035-46 (2010)

2010
727
The making of hemidesmosome structures in vivo.
[20205195] Dev Dyn 239(5):1465-76 (2010)

2010
728
Evolution of programmed cell fusion: common mechanisms and distinct functions.
[20419783] Dev Dyn 239(5):1515-28 (2010)

2008
729
The primary cilium as a gravitational force transducer and a regulator of transcriptional noise.
[18366139] Dev Dyn 237(8):1955-9 (2008)

2008
730
Assembly of primary cilia.
[18393310] Dev Dyn 237(8):1993-2006 (2008)

2008
731
Building it up and taking it down: the regulation of vertebrate ciliogenesis.
[18435467] Dev Dyn 237(8):1972-81 (2008)

2003
732
Changes in spinal cord regenerative ability through phylogenesis and development: lessons to be learnt.
[12557203] Dev Dyn 226(2):245-56 (2003)

2003
733
Cnidarians: an evolutionarily conserved model system for regeneration?
[12557204] Dev Dyn 226(2):257-67 (2003)

2003
734
Regeneration or scarring: an immunologic perspective.
[12557205] Dev Dyn 226(2):268-79 (2003)

2003
735
Regeneration of the urodele limb: a review.
[12557206] Dev Dyn 226(2):280-94 (2003)

2003
736
Urodele spinal cord regeneration and related processes.
[12557207] Dev Dyn 226(2):295-307 (2003)

2003   **Intercalary regeneration in planarians.**
737   [12557208] Dev Dyn 226(2):308-16 (2003)

2003   **Pronephric duct extension in amphibian embryos: migration and other mechanisms.**
738   [12508219] Dev Dyn 226(1):1-11 (2003)

2003   **Muscle regeneration in amphibians and mammals: passing the torch.**
739   [12557196] Dev Dyn 226(2):167-81 (2003)

2003   **Hydra regeneration and epitheliopeptides.**
740   [12557197] Dev Dyn 226(2):182-9 (2003)

2003   **Old questions, new tools, and some answers to the mystery of fin regeneration.**
741   [12557198] Dev Dyn 226(2):190-201 (2003)

2003   **Tales of regeneration in zebrafish.**
742   [12557199] Dev Dyn 226(2):202-10 (2003)

2003   **Eye regeneration at the molecular age.**
743   [12557200] Dev Dyn 226(2):211-24 (2003)

2003   **Head regeneration in Hydra.**
744   [12557201] Dev Dyn 226(2):225-36 (2003)

2008   **MAP3Ks as central regulators of cell fate during development.**
745   [18855897] Dev Dyn 237(11):3102-14 (2008)

2007   **Back to basics: Sox genes.**
746   [17584862] Dev Dyn 236(8):2356-66 (2007)

2007   **Hox patterning of the vertebrate axial skeleton.**
747   [17685480] Dev Dyn 236(9):2454-63 (2007)

2009   **In vitro organogenesis from undifferentiated cells in Xenopus.**
748   [19441056] Dev Dyn 238(6):1309-20 (2009)

2006   **Mathematical model of morphogen electrophoresis through gap junctions.**
749   [16786594] Dev Dyn 235(8):2144-59 (2006)

2010   **Mass spectrometry-based metabolomics, analysis of metabolite-protein interactions, and imaging.**
750   [20701590] Biotechniques 49(2):557-65 (2010)

2011   **Mitochondrial membrane potential probes and the proton gradient: a practical usage guide.**
751   [21486251] Biotechniques 50(2):98-115 (2011)

2011   **Label-free analysis of biomolecular interactions using SPR imaging.**
752   [21231920] Biotechniques 50(1):32-40 (2011)

2011   **Modern fluorescent proteins: from chromophore formation to novel intracellular applications.**
753   [22054544] Biotechniques 51(5):313-4, 316, 318 passim (2011)

2011   **Tissue engineering tools for modulation of the immune response.**
754   [21988690] Biotechniques 51(4):239-40, 242, 244 passim (2011)

2010   **Advances in genome-wide DNA methylation analysis.**
755   [20964631] Biotechniques 49(4):iii-xi (2010)

2010   **Antibody validation.**
756   [20359301] Biotechniques 48(3):197-209 (2010)

2009
757
ALISSA: an automated live-cell imaging system for signal transduction analyses.
[20041856] Biotechniques 47(6):1033-40 (2009)

2007
758
Potential solutions for confocal imaging of living animals.
[17933097] Biotechniques 43(1 Suppl):14-9 (2007)

2007
759
Building a dynamic fate map.
[17933098] Biotechniques 43(1 Suppl):20-4 (2007)

2007
760
Validity of bioluminescence measurements for noninvasive in vivo imaging of tumor load in small animals.
[17936938] Biotechniques 43(1 Suppl):7-13, 30 (2007)

2007
761
Electron cryotomography.
[18019332] Biotechniques 43(4):413, 415, 417 passim (2007)

2005
762
Disposable microfluidic devices: fabrication, function, and application.
[15786809] Biotechniques 38(3):429-46 (2005)

2005
763
Enzymatic mutation detection technologies.
[15948293] Biotechniques 38(5):749-58 (2005)

2009
764
Genome sequence data: management, storage, and visualization.
[19480628] Biotechniques 46(5):333-4, 336 (2009)

2009
765
Extracting evidence from forensic DNA analyses: future molecular biology directions.
[19480629] Biotechniques 46(5):339-40, 342-50 (2009)

2009
766
Self-reporting cells.
[19480631] Biotechniques 46(5):356-7 (2009)

2005
767
Spectral domain optical coherence tomography: a better OCT imaging strategy.
[20158503] Biotechniques 39(6 Suppl):S6-13 (2005)

2008
768
Kits and their unique role in molecular biology: a brief retrospective.
[18474048] Biotechniques 44(5):701-4 (2008)

2008
769
Two-dimensional polyacrylamide gel electrophoresis (2D-PAGE): advances and perspectives.
[18474047] Biotechniques 44(5):697-8, 700 (2008)

2008
770
Epitope tagging.
[18474046] Biotechniques 44(5):693-5 (2008)

2008
771
Interactive proteomics: what lies ahead?
[18474045] Biotechniques 44(5):681-91 (2008)

2008
772
The evolution of tools for protein phosphorylation site analysis: from discovery to clinical application.
[18474044] Biotechniques 44(5):671-9 (2008)

2008
773
Hexapeptide combinatorial ligand libraries: the march for the detection of the low-abundance proteome continues.
[18474042] Biotechniques 44(5):663-5 (2008)

2008
774
Resolving the network of cell signaling pathways using the evolving yeast two-hybrid system.
[18474041] Biotechniques 44(5):655-62 (2008)

2008
775
Deep cap analysis gene expression (CAGE): genome-wide identification of promoters, quantification of their expression, and network inference.
[18474037] Biotechniques 44(5):627-8, 630, 632 (2008)

2008   **RNAi mechanisms and applications.**
776   [18474035] Biotechniques 44(5):613-6 (2008)

2008   **FISH glossary: an overview of the fluorescence in situ hybridization technique.**
777   [18855767] Biotechniques 45(4):385-6, 388, 390 passim (2008)

2005   **Real-time PCR for mRNA quantitation.**
778   [16060372] Biotechniques 39(1):75-85 (2005)

2005   **Mammalian RNAi: a practical guide.**
779   [16116795] Biotechniques 39(2):215-24 (2005)

2006   **Analysis of posttranslational modifications of proteins by tandem mass spectrometry.**
780   [16774123] Biotechniques 40(6):790-8 (2006)

2011   **Controversies in clinical cancer dormancy.**
781   [21746894] Proc Natl Acad Sci U S A 108(30):12396-400 (2011)

2002   **Quantum dot artificial solids: understanding the static and dynamic role of size and packing disorder.**
782   [11880611] Proc Natl Acad Sci U S A 99 Suppl 2(-):6456-9 (2002)

2010   **MiDReG: a method of mining developmentally regulated genes using Boolean implications.**
783   [20231483] Proc Natl Acad Sci U S A 107(13):5732-7 (2010)

2003   **Cancer risks attributable to low doses of ionizing radiation: assessing what we really know.**
784   [14610281] Proc Natl Acad Sci U S A 100(24):13761-6 (2003)

2003   **Electron-nuclear double resonance spectroscopy (and electron spin-echo envelope modulation spectroscopy) in bioinorganic chemistry.**
785   [12642664] Proc Natl Acad Sci U S A 100(7):3575-8 (2003)

2003   **New clues for platinum antitumor chemistry: kinetically controlled metal binding to DNA.**
786   [12655051] Proc Natl Acad Sci U S A 100(7):3611-6 (2003)

2003   **Biological inorganic chemistry at the beginning of the 21st century.**
787   [12657732] Proc Natl Acad Sci U S A 100(7):3563-8 (2003)

2008   **Geomagnetic imprinting: A unifying hypothesis of long-distance natal homing in salmon and sea turtles.**
788   [19060188] Proc Natl Acad Sci U S A 105(49):19096-101 (2008)

2007   **Exceptionally well preserved late Quaternary plant and vertebrate fossils from a blue hole on Abaco, The Bahamas.**
789   [18077421] Proc Natl Acad Sci U S A 104(50):19897-902 (2007)

2005   **Logic functions of the genomic cis-regulatory code.**
790   [15788531] Proc Natl Acad Sci U S A 102(14):4954-9 (2005)

2005   **The rise of the ants: a phylogenetic and ecological explanation.**
791   [15899976] Proc Natl Acad Sci U S A 102(21):7411-4 (2005)

2009   **Genome-wide association and meta-analysis of bipolar disorder in individuals of European ancestry.**
792   [19416921] Proc Natl Acad Sci U S A 106(18):7501-6 (2009)

2009   **Hsp90 inhibitor PU-H71, a multimodal inhibitor of malignancy, induces complete responses in triple-negative breast cancer models.**
793   [19416831] Proc Natl Acad Sci U S A 106(20):8368-73 (2009)

2008   **Variation in virulence among clades of Escherichia coli O157:H7 associated with disease outbreaks.**
794   [18332430] Proc Natl Acad Sci U S A 105(12):4868-73 (2008)

2009
795

Endosomes: a legitimate platform for the signaling train.
[19822761] Proc Natl Acad Sci U S A 106(42):17615-22 (2009)

2009
796

The genetic architecture of Down syndrome phenotypes revealed by high-resolution analysis of human segmental trisomies.
[19597142] Proc Natl Acad Sci U S A 106(29):12031-6 (2009)

2010
797

Examining the case for the effect of barrier compression on tunneling, vibrationally enhanced catalysis, catalytic entropy and related issues.
[20433839] FEBS Lett 584(13):2759-66 (2010)

2010
798

NPC1L1 and cholesterol transport.
[20307540] FEBS Lett 584(13):2740-7 (2010)

2010
799

The mitochondrial permeability transition from yeast to mammals.
[20398660] FEBS Lett 584(12):2504-9 (2010)

2010
800

TPCs: Endolysosomal channels for Ca2+ mobilization from acidic organelles triggered by NAADP.
[20159015] FEBS Lett 584(10):1966-74 (2010)

2010
801

Sphingomyelin metabolism at the plasma membrane: implications for bioactive sphingolipids.
[19857494] FEBS Lett 584(9):1887-94 (2010)

2009
802

Spatially distributed cell signalling.
[19800332] FEBS Lett 583(24):4006-12 (2009)

2010
803

Chaperone-mediated autophagy in health and disease.
[20026330] FEBS Lett 584(7):1399-404 (2010)

2010
804

Cellular dynamics of tRNAs and their genes.
[19931532] FEBS Lett 584(2):310-7 (2010)

2010
805

Unexpected diversity of RNase P, an ancient tRNA processing enzyme: challenges and prospects.
[19931535] FEBS Lett 584(2):287-96 (2010)

2010
806

The T box mechanism: tRNA as a regulatory molecule.
[19932103] FEBS Lett 584(2):318-24 (2010)

2010
807

The balance between pre- and post-transfer editing in tRNA synthetases.
[19941860] FEBS Lett 584(2):455-9 (2010)

2010
808

Stereochemical mechanisms of tRNA methyltransferases.
[19944101] FEBS Lett 584(2):278-86 (2010)

2010
809

Chloride channels of intracellular membranes.
[20100480] FEBS Lett 584(10):2102-11 (2010)

2010
810

Molecular mechanism and physiological role of pexophagy.
[20083110] FEBS Lett 584(7):1367-73 (2010)

2010
811

mTOR regulation of autophagy.
[20083114] FEBS Lett 584(7):1287-95 (2010)

2010
812

Autophagy in cellular growth control.
[20096689] FEBS Lett 584(7):1417-26 (2010)

2010
813

Parkin-mediated selective mitochondrial autophagy, mitophagy: Parkin purges damaged organelles from the vital mitochondrial network.
[20188730] FEBS Lett 584(7):1386-92 (2010)

2010 **tRNAs: cellular barcodes for amino acids.**
814 [19903480] FEBS Lett 584(2):387-95 (2010)

2010 **Eukaryotic initiator tRNA: finely tuned and ready for action.**
815 [19925799] FEBS Lett 584(2):396-404 (2010)

2009 **Glycoproteomics: past, present and future.**
816 [19328791] FEBS Lett 583(11):1728-35 (2009)

2008 **RNA-binding proteins and post-transcriptional gene regulation.**
817 [18342629] FEBS Lett 582(14):1977-86 (2008)

2008 **Lipid rafts and T-lymphocyte function: implications for autoimmunity.**
818 [18930053] FEBS Lett 582(27):3711-8 (2008)

2009 **Role of vesicle tethering factors in the ER-Golgi membrane traffic.**
819 [19887069] FEBS Lett 583(23):3770-83 (2009)

2009 **Positive-feedback loops in cell cycle progression.**
820 [19818353] FEBS Lett 583(21):3388-96 (2009)

2009 **The yeast Golgi apparatus: insights and mysteries.**
821 [19879270] FEBS Lett 583(23):3746-51 (2009)

2009 **Multiple routes of protein transport from endosomes to the trans Golgi network.**
822 [19879268] FEBS Lett 583(23):3811-6 (2009)

2009 **Animal models of human amyloidoses: are transgenic mice worth the time and trouble?**
823 [19627988] FEBS Lett 583(16):2663-73 (2009)

2010 **Viral miRNAs: tools for immune evasion.**
824 [20580307] Curr Opin Microbiol 13(4):540-5 (2010)

2010 **Studying bacterial transcriptomes using RNA-seq.**
825 [20888288] Curr Opin Microbiol 13(5):619-24 (2010)

2010 **Sensor domains of two-component regulatory systems.**
826 [20223701] Curr Opin Microbiol 13(2):116-23 (2010)

2010 **Receiver domain structure and function in response regulator proteins.**
827 [20211578] Curr Opin Microbiol 13(2):142-9 (2010)

2010 **Two-component signal transduction.**
828 [20219418] Curr Opin Microbiol 13(2):113-5 (2010)

2008 **Leishmania sand fly interaction: progress and challenges.**
829 [18625337] Curr Opin Microbiol 11(4):340-4 (2008)

2010 **Auxiliary phosphatases in two-component signal transduction.**
830 [20133180] Curr Opin Microbiol 13(2):177-83 (2010)

2010 **Interaction fidelity in two-component signaling.**
831 [20133181] Curr Opin Microbiol 13(2):190-7 (2010)

2010 **Two-component signaling circuit structure and properties.**
832 [20149717] Curr Opin Microbiol 13(2):184-9 (2010)

2010 **Orphan and hybrid two-component system proteins in health and disease.**
833 [20089442] Curr Opin Microbiol 13(2):226-31 (2010)

2010   Physiologically relevant small phosphodonors link metabolism to signal transduction.
834   [20117041] Curr Opin Microbiol 13(2):204-9 (2010)

2010   Bacterial chemoreceptors: providing enhanced features to two-component signaling.
835   [20122866] Curr Opin Microbiol 13(2):124-32 (2010)

2007   Is phage DNA 'injected' into cells--biologists and physicists can agree.
836   [17714979] Curr Opin Microbiol 10(4):401-9 (2007)

2007   Antibiotic resistant Staphylococcus aureus: a paradigm of adaptive power.
837   [17921044] Curr Opin Microbiol 10(5):428-35 (2007)

2007   Overview of cell shape: cytoskeletons shape bacterial cells.
838   [17980647] Curr Opin Microbiol 10(6):601-5 (2007)

2007   Encystation of Giardia lamblia: a model for other parasites.
839   [17981075] Curr Opin Microbiol 10(6):554-9 (2007)

2007   Bacterial morphology: why have different shapes?
840   [17981076] Curr Opin Microbiol 10(6):596-600 (2007)

2007   Thinking about Bacillus subtilis as a multicellular organism.
841   [17977783] Curr Opin Microbiol 10(6):638-43 (2007)

2007   Role of polysaccharides in Pseudomonas aeruginosa biofilm development.
842   [17981495] Curr Opin Microbiol 10(6):644-8 (2007)

2007   Rhoptries: an arsenal of secreted virulence factors.
843   [17997128] Curr Opin Microbiol 10(6):582-7 (2007)

2009   New developments in microbial interspecies signaling.
844   [19251475] Curr Opin Microbiol 12(2):205-14 (2009)

2008   Ionizing radiation: how fungi cope, adapt, and exploit with the help of melanin.
845   [18848901] Curr Opin Microbiol 11(6):525-31 (2008)

2007   The intricate world of riboswitches.
846   [17383225] Curr Opin Microbiol 10(2):176-81 (2007)

2009   Electron cryotomography: a new view into microbial ultrastructure.
847   [19427259] Curr Opin Microbiol 12(3):333-40 (2009)

2009   Mechanisms of hypha orientation of fungi.
848   [19546023] Curr Opin Microbiol 12(4):350-7 (2009)

2008   Therapeutic potential of type A (I) lantibiotics, a group of cationic peptide antibiotics.
849   [18848642] Curr Opin Microbiol 11(5):401-8 (2008)

2008   Bacteriophage lysins as effective antibacterials.
850   [18824123] Curr Opin Microbiol 11(5):393-400 (2008)

2008   Fungal killing by mammalian phagocytic cells.
851   [18573683] Curr Opin Microbiol 11(4):313-7 (2008)

2005   Bridging the imaging gap: visualizing subcellular architecture with electron tomography.
852   [15939356] Curr Opin Microbiol 8(3):316-22 (2005)

2009   Plasmodium sporozoite-host interactions from the dermis to the hepatocyte.
853   [19608456] Curr Opin Microbiol 12(4):401-7 (2009)

2002   **The shikimate pathway and its branches in apicomplexan parasites.**
854   [11865437] J Infect Dis 185 Suppl 1(-):S25-36 (2002)

2010   **Clinical management of acute HIV infection: best practice remains unknown.**
855   [20846034] J Infect Dis 202 Suppl 2(-):S278-88 (2010)

2010   **The detection of acute HIV infection.**
856   [20846033] J Infect Dis 202 Suppl 2(-):S270-7 (2010)

2010   **Advantages of peptide nucleic acids as diagnostic platforms for detection of nucleic acids in resource-limited settings.**
857   [20225945] J Infect Dis 201 Suppl 1(-):S42-5 (2010)

2005   **A vaccine-preventable infectious disease kills half a million children annually.**
858   [16235162] J Infect Dis 192(10):1679-80 (2005)

2004   **The clinical significance of measles: a review.**
859   [15106083] J Infect Dis 189 Suppl 1(-):S4-16 (2004)

2004   **Ebola virus ecology.**
860   [15529250] J Infect Dis 190(11):1893-4 (2004)

2004   **Simian virus 40 and human disease.**
861   [15551202] J Infect Dis 190(12):2061-4 (2004)

2003   **Ebola hemorrhagic fever and septic shock.**
862   [14639530] J Infect Dis 188(11):1613-7 (2003)

2008   **Immunodominance and recognition of intracellular pathogens.**
863   [18922096] J Infect Dis 198(11):1579-81 (2008)

2007   **The 1918 influenza pandemic: insights for the 21st century.**
864   [17330793] J Infect Dis 195(7):1018-28 (2007)

2008   **Practical consequences of hepatitis C virus quasispecies for target-specific antivirals.**
865   [18637751] J Infect Dis 198(6):797-9 (2008)

2011   **Intracellular events and cell fate in filovirus infection.**
866   [21927676] Viruses 3(8):1501-31 (2011)

2011   **Converging strategies in expression of human complex retroviruses.**
867   [21994786] Viruses 3(8):1395-414 (2011)

2011   **Recombination between poliovirus and coxsackie A viruses of species C: a model of viral genetic plasticity and emergence.**
868   [21994791] Viruses 3(8):1460-84 (2011)

2011   **The role of interferon antagonist, non-structural proteins in the pathogenesis and emergence of arboviruses.**
869   [21994750] Viruses 3(6):629-58 (2011)

2011   **CD4+ T cell depletion in human immunodeficiency virus (HIV) infection: role of apoptosis.**
870   [21994747] Viruses 3(5):586-612 (2011)

2011   **Insertional oncogenesis by non-acute retroviruses: implications for gene therapy.**
871   [21994739] Viruses 3(4):398-422 (2011)

2011   **Bacteriophage assembly.**
872   [21994726] Viruses 3(3):172-203 (2011)

2011   Antiviral inhibition of enveloped virus release by tetherin/BST-2: action and counteraction.
873   [21994744] Viruses 3(5):520-40 (2011)

2011   Next generation sequencing technologies for insect virus discovery.
874   [22069519] Viruses 3(10):1849-69 (2011)

2011   Viral ancestors of antiviral systems.
875   [22069523] Viruses 3(10):1933-58 (2011)

2011   The molecular biology of frog virus 3 and other iridoviruses infecting cold-blooded vertebrates.
876   [22069524] Viruses 3(10):1959-85 (2011)

2010   T cell polarization at the virological synapse.
877   [21994679] Viruses 2(6):1261-78 (2010)

2010   Pathogenesis of noroviruses, emerging RNA viruses.
878   [21994656] Viruses 2(3):748-81 (2010)

2010   HIV-1 Virological Synapse is not Simply a Copycat of the Immunological Synapse.
879   [20890395] Viruses 2(5):1239-60 (2010)

2010   RNA replicons - a new approach for influenza virus immunoprophylaxis.
880   [21994644] Viruses 2(2):413-34 (2010)

2002   Clinical aspects and pathophysiology of inflammatory bowel disease.
881   [11781268] Clin Microbiol Rev 15(1):79-94 (2002)

2002   Modulation of release of proinflammatory bacterial compounds by antibacterials: potential impact
882   on course of inflammation and outcome in sepsis and meningitis.
   [11781269] Clin Microbiol Rev 15(1):95-110 (2002)

2002   Interactions among strategies associated with bacterial infection: pathogenicity, epidemicity, and
883   antibiotic resistance.
   [12364374] Clin Microbiol Rev 15(4):647-79 (2002)

2010   Community-associated methicillin-resistant Staphylococcus aureus: epidemiology and clinical
884   consequences of an emerging epidemic.
   [20610826] Clin Microbiol Rev 23(3):616-87 (2010)

2010   Epidemiology, treatment, and prevention of human T-cell leukemia virus type 1-associated diseases.
885   [20610824] Clin Microbiol Rev 23(3):577-89 (2010)

2010   The changing epidemiology of Clostridium difficile infections.
886   [20610822] Clin Microbiol Rev 23(3):529-49 (2010)

2010   Medical and legal implications of testing for sexually transmitted infections in children.
887   [20610820] Clin Microbiol Rev 23(3):493-506 (2010)

2010   Epidemiology, diagnosis, and antimicrobial treatment of acute bacterial meningitis.
888   [20610819] Clin Microbiol Rev 23(3):467-92 (2010)

2010   Role of bacteria in oncogenesis.
889   [20930075] Clin Microbiol Rev 23(4):837-57 (2010)

2010   Penetration of drugs through the blood-cerebrospinal fluid/blood-brain barrier for treatment of
890   central nervous system infections.
   [20930076] Clin Microbiol Rev 23(4):858-83 (2010)

2010   Antiviral drug resistance of human cytomegalovirus.
891   [20930070] Clin Microbiol Rev 23(4):689-712 (2010)

2010
892   Helicobacter pylori and gastric cancer: factors that modulate disease risk.
[20930071] Clin Microbiol Rev 23(4):713-39 (2010)

2010
893   Infections of people with complement deficiencies and patients who have undergone splenectomy.
[20930072] Clin Microbiol Rev 23(4):740-80 (2010)

2010
894   Molecular pathogenesis of infections caused by Legionella pneumophila.
[20375353] Clin Microbiol Rev 23(2):274-98 (2010)

2010
895   The changing microbial epidemiology in cystic fibrosis.
[20375354] Clin Microbiol Rev 23(2):299-323 (2010)

2010
896   Cardiac involvement with parasitic infections.
[20375355] Clin Microbiol Rev 23(2):324-49 (2010)

2010
897   Clinical and laboratory update on blastomycosis.
[20375357] Clin Microbiol Rev 23(2):367-81 (2010)

2010
898   Epidemiology of seafood-associated infections in the United States.
[20375359] Clin Microbiol Rev 23(2):399-411 (2010)

2010
899   A global perspective on hantavirus ecology, epidemiology, and disease.
[20375360] Clin Microbiol Rev 23(2):412-41 (2010)

2010
900   The era of molecular and other non-culture-based methods in diagnosis of sepsis.
[20065332] Clin Microbiol Rev 23(1):235-51 (2010)

2010
901   Rifampin combination therapy for nonmycobacterial infections.
[20065324] Clin Microbiol Rev 23(1):14-34 (2010)

2010
902   The genus Aeromonas: taxonomy, pathogenicity, and infection.
[20065325] Clin Microbiol Rev 23(1):35-73 (2010)

2010
903   Respiratory viral infections in infants: causes, clinical symptoms, virology, and immunology.
[20065326] Clin Microbiol Rev 23(1):74-98 (2010)

2010
904   Three decades of beta-lactamase inhibitors.
[20065329] Clin Microbiol Rev 23(1):160-201 (2010)

2007
905   Ventilator-associated pneumonia in neonatal and pediatric intensive care unit patients.
[17630332] Clin Microbiol Rev 20(3):409-25, table of contents (2007)

2009
906   Matrix metalloproteinases as drug targets in infections caused by gram-negative bacteria and in septic shock.
[19366913] Clin Microbiol Rev 22(2):224-39, Table of Contents (2009)

2005
907   Current and developing technologies for monitoring agents of bioterrorism and biowarfare.
[16223949] Clin Microbiol Rev 18(4):583-607 (2005)

2005
908   Biological transmission of arboviruses: reexamination of and new insights into components, mechanisms, and unique traits as well as their evolutionary trends.
[16223950] Clin Microbiol Rev 18(4):608-37 (2005)

2008
909   Respiratory viruses other than influenza virus: impact and therapeutic advances.
[18400797] Clin Microbiol Rev 21(2):274-90, table of contents (2008)

2008
910   New insights on classification, identification, and clinical relevance of Blastocystis spp.
[18854485] Clin Microbiol Rev 21(4):639-65 (2008)

2008
911

Emergence and disappearance of a virulent clone of Haemophilus influenzae biogroup aegyptius, cause of Brazilian purpuric fever.
[18854482] Clin Microbiol Rev 21(4):594-605 (2008)

2005
912

Enterotoxigenic Escherichia coli in developing countries: epidemiology, microbiology, clinical features, treatment, and prevention.
[16020685] Clin Microbiol Rev 18(3):465-83 (2005)

2009
913

Immune restoration diseases reflect diverse immunopathological mechanisms.
[19822893] Clin Microbiol Rev 22(4):651-63 (2009)

2009
914

Antibacterial-resistant Pseudomonas aeruginosa: clinical impact and complex regulation of chromosomally encoded resistance mechanisms.
[19822890] Clin Microbiol Rev 22(4):582-610 (2009)

2009
915

Dengue virus pathogenesis: an integrated view.
[19822889] Clin Microbiol Rev 22(4):564-81 (2009)

2009
916

Modern uses of electron microscopy for detection of viruses.
[19822888] Clin Microbiol Rev 22(4):552-63 (2009)

2009
917

Food-borne trematodiases.
[19597009] Clin Microbiol Rev 22(3):466-83 (2009)

2009
918

Pathogenesis of Aspergillus fumigatus in Invasive Aspergillosis.
[19597008] Clin Microbiol Rev 22(3):447-65 (2009)

2009
919

North American paragonimiasis (Caused by Paragonimus kellicotti) in the context of global paragonimiasis.
[19597007] Clin Microbiol Rev 22(3):415-46 (2009)

2009
920

Pathogenesis, diagnosis, and management of primary antibody deficiencies and infections.
[19597006] Clin Microbiol Rev 22(3):396-414 (2009)

2008
921

Transmission of tropical and geographically restricted infections during solid-organ transplantation.
[18202437] Clin Microbiol Rev 21(1):60-96 (2008)

2010
922

The difficulty of targeting cancer stem cell niches.
[20530700] Clin Cancer Res 16(12):3121-9 (2010)

2010
923

Fluorescence resonance energy transfer biosensors for cancer detection and evaluation of drug efficacy.
[20670948] Clin Cancer Res 16(15):3822-4 (2010)

2011
924

ERK1/2 and p38α/β² signaling in tumor cell quiescence: opportunities to control dormant residual disease.
[21673068] Clin Cancer Res 17(18):5850-7 (2011)

2010
925

Metformin: a therapeutic opportunity in breast cancer.
[20215559] Clin Cancer Res 16(6):1695-700 (2010)

2004
926

Reanalysis of cancer drugs: old drugs, new tricks.
[15173099] Clin Cancer Res 10(11):3897-907 (2004)

2004
927

Mammalian target of rapamycin inhibition.
[15448035] Clin Cancer Res 10(18 Pt 2):6382S-7S (2004)

2004
928

Use of replicating oncolytic adenoviruses in combination therapy for cancer.
[15328165] Clin Cancer Res 10(16):5299-312 (2004)

| 2003 | **NLCQ-1 (NSC 709257): exploiting hypoxia with a weak DNA-intercalating bioreductive drug.** |
| 929 | [14654556] Clin Cancer Res 9(15):5714-20 (2003) |

| 2003 | **Soft tissue sarcomas of adults: state of the translational science.** |
| 930 | [12796356] Clin Cancer Res 9(6):1941-56 (2003) |

| 2008 | **Microtubule active agents: beyond the taxane frontier.** |
| 931 | [19010832] Clin Cancer Res 14(22):7167-72 (2008) |

| 2010 | **Nuclear factor-kappaB and tumor-associated macrophages.** |
| 932 | [20103670] Clin Cancer Res 16(3):784-9 (2010) |

| 2007 | **PD-1 is expressed by tumor-infiltrating immune cells and is associated with poor outcome for patients with renal cell carcinoma.** |
| 933 | [17363529] Clin Cancer Res 13(6):1757-61 (2007) |

| 2007 | **Whole-body optical imaging in animal models to assess cancer development and progression.** |
| 934 | [17575211] Clin Cancer Res 13(12):3490-7 (2007) |

| 2005 | **Cell death independent of caspases: a review.** |
| 935 | [15867207] Clin Cancer Res 11(9):3155-62 (2005) |

| 2008 | **Capitalizing on the immunogenicity of dying tumor cells.** |
| 936 | [18347160] Clin Cancer Res 14(6):1603-8 (2008) |

| 2008 | **Validation of analytic methods for biomarkers used in drug development.** |
| 937 | [18829475] Clin Cancer Res 14(19):5967-76 (2008) |

| 2009 | **Lysine 63 polyubiquitination in immunotherapy and in cancer-promoting inflammation.** |
| 938 | [19887490] Clin Cancer Res 15(22):6751-7 (2009) |

| 2009 | **MYC-induced cancer cell energy metabolism and therapeutic opportunities.** |
| 939 | [19861459] Clin Cancer Res 15(21):6479-83 (2009) |

| 2009 | **The multifaceted role of MTDH/AEG-1 in cancer progression.** |
| 940 | [19723648] Clin Cancer Res 15(18):5615-20 (2009) |

| 2009 | **Disrupting polyamine homeostasis as a therapeutic strategy for neuroblastoma.** |
| 941 | [19789308] Clin Cancer Res 15(19):5956-61 (2009) |

| 2009 | **Heat shock protein 90 as a drug target: some like it hot.** |
| 942 | [19118027] Clin Cancer Res 15(1):9-14 (2009) |

| 2002 | **Impact of tumor hypoxia and anemia on radiation therapy outcomes.** |
| 943 | [12490737] Oncologist 7(6):492-508 (2002) |

| 2010 | **Radioprotectors and mitigators of radiation-induced normal tissue injury.** |
| 944 | [20413641] Oncologist 15(4):360-71 (2010) |

| 2010 | **High-intensity focused ultrasound in the treatment of bone tumors: another treatment option for palliation and primary treatment?** |
| 945 | [20564114] Cancer 116(16):3754-5 (2010) |

| 2010 | **Development of curcumin as an epigenetic agent.** |
| 946 | [20597137] Cancer 116(20):4670-6 (2010) |

| 2010 | **Tumor progression by immune evasion in melanoma: role of the programmed cell death-1/programmed cell death-1 ligand 1 interaction.** |
| 947 | [20143442] Cancer 116(7):1623-5 (2010) |

2010 Disrupting established tumor blood vessels: an emerging therapeutic strategy for cancer.
948   [20166210] Cancer 116(8):1859-71 (2010)

2009 Bayesian statistics in oncology: a guide for the clinical investigator.
949   [19691089] Cancer 115(23):5371-81 (2009)

2010 Tipping the balance: Cdk2 enables Myc to suppress senescence.
950   [20713526] Cancer Res 70(17):6687-91 (2010)

2010 CD73: a novel target for cancer immunotherapy.
951   [20682793] Cancer Res 70(16):6407-11 (2010)

2010 Monitoring of natural killer cell immunotherapy using noninvasive imaging modalities.
952   [20631071] Cancer Res 70(15):6109-13 (2010)

2006 Distinct role of macrophages in different tumor microenvironments.
953   [16423985] Cancer Res 66(2):605-12 (2006)

2006 Normal stem cells and cancer stem cells: the niche matters.
954   [16651403] Cancer Res 66(9):4553-7 (2006)

2006 Exploring a new twist on tumor metastasis.
955   [16651402] Cancer Res 66(9):4549-52 (2006)

2006 The DNA damage response arouses the immune system.
956   [16618710] Cancer Res 66(8):3959-62 (2006)

2006 Lysyl oxidase mediates hypoxic control of metastasis.
957   [17079439] Cancer Res 66(21):10238-41 (2006)

2006 Quantitating therapeutic disruption of tumor blood flow with intravital video microscopy.
958   [17178842] Cancer Res 66(24):11517-9 (2006)

2010 AACR special conference on epithelial-mesenchymal transition and cancer progression and
959   treatment.
       [20823151] Cancer Res 70(19):7360-4 (2010)

2010 Cancer stem cells in the central nervous system--a critical review.
960   [20959482] Cancer Res 70(21):8255-8 (2010)

2010 Turning on a fuel switch of cancer: hnRNP proteins regulate alternative splicing of pyruvate kinase
961   mRNA.
       [20978194] Cancer Res 70(22):8977-80 (2010)

2010 An ex(o)citing machinery for invasive tumor growth.
962   [21098711] Cancer Res 70(23):9533-7 (2010)

2010 Mammalian target of rapamycin activator RHEB is frequently overexpressed in human carcinomas
963   and is critical and sufficient for skin epithelial carcinogenesis.
       [20388784] Cancer Res 70(8):3287-98 (2010)

2010 Immune promotion of epithelial-mesenchymal transition and generation of breast cancer stem cells.
964   [20395197] Cancer Res 70(8):3005-8 (2010)

2010 Telomere loss as a mechanism for chromosome instability in human cancer.
965   [20484032] Cancer Res 70(11):4255-9 (2010)

2010 Drugging the PI3 kinome: from chemical tools to drugs in the clinic.
966   [20179189] Cancer Res 70(6):2146-57 (2010)

2010
967
Intravital imaging illuminates transforming growth factor beta signaling switches during metastasis.
[20424121] Cancer Res 70(9):3435-9 (2010)

2004
968
Modern criteria to establish human cancer etiology.
[15289363] Cancer Res 64(15):5518-24 (2004)

2009
969
Mutant metabolic enzymes are at the origin of gliomas.
[19996293] Cancer Res 69(24):9157-9 (2009)

2010
970
The nicotinamide phosphoribosyltransferase: a molecular link between metabolism, inflammation, and cancer.
[20028851] Cancer Res 70(1):8-11 (2010)

2003
971
The days and nights of cancer cells.
[14633665] Cancer Res 63(22):7545-52 (2003)

2010
972
Dendritic cell-derived exosomes for cancer immunotherapy: what's next?
[20145139] Cancer Res 70(4):1281-5 (2010)

2010
973
Defective mismatch repair, microsatellite mutation bias, and variability in clinical cancer phenotypes.
[20068152] Cancer Res 70(2):431-5 (2010)

2010
974
Rethinking the Warburg effect with Myc micromanaging glutamine metabolism.
[20086171] Cancer Res 70(3):859-62 (2010)

2007
975
Antiangiogenic strategies on defense: on the possibility of blocking rebounds by the tumor vasculature after chemotherapy.
[17671170] Cancer Res 67(15):7055-8 (2007)

2007
976
Tumor angiogenesis: cause or consequence of cancer?
[17671171] Cancer Res 67(15):7059-61 (2007)

2007
977
4E-binding protein 1: a key molecular "funnel factor" in human cancer with clinical implications.
[17699757] Cancer Res 67(16):7551-5 (2007)

2007
978
Tie2-expressing monocytes and tumor angiogenesis: regulation by hypoxia and angiopoietin-2.
[17875679] Cancer Res 67(18):8429-32 (2007)

2007
979
A new central scaffold for metastasis: parsing HEF1/Cas-L/NEDD9.
[17908996] Cancer Res 67(19):8975-9 (2007)

2007
980
Leveraging the immune system during chemotherapy: moving calreticulin to the cell surface converts apoptotic death from "silent" to immunogenic.
[17804698] Cancer Res 67(17):7941-4 (2007)

2007
981
Regulation of mTOR by phosphatidic acid?
[17210675] Cancer Res 67(1):1-4 (2007)

2007
982
Notch signaling, gamma-secretase inhibitors, and cancer therapy.
[17332312] Cancer Res 67(5):1879-82 (2007)

2007
983
Genome-wide, high-resolution detection of copy number, loss of heterozygosity, and genotypes from formalin-fixed, paraffin-embedded tumor tissue using microarrays.
[17363572] Cancer Res 67(6):2544-51 (2007)

2009
984
Cancer prevention: from 1727 to milestones of the past 100 years.
[19491253] Cancer Res 69(13):5269-84 (2009)

2009
985
Aurora-A and hBora join the game of Polo.
[19487276] Cancer Res 69(11):4555-8 (2009)

2009
986
Antitumor activity with CYP17 blockade indicates that castration-resistant prostate cancer frequently remains hormone driven.
[19509232] Cancer Res 69(12):4937-40 (2009)

2009
987
Therapeutic potential of "rexinoids" in cancer prevention and treatment.
[19509234] Cancer Res 69(12):4945-7 (2009)

2009
988
Unwelcome complement.
[19654288] Cancer Res 69(16):6367-70 (2009)

2005
989
The transcription factor Pokemon: a new key player in cancer pathogenesis.
[16204018] Cancer Res 65(19):8575-8 (2005)

2008
990
Tumor-specific T-cell memory: clearing the regulatory T-cell hurdle.
[18339838] Cancer Res 68(6):1614-7 (2008)

2008
991
Role of the aggresome pathway in cancer: targeting histone deacetylase 6-dependent protein degradation.
[18413721] Cancer Res 68(8):2557-60 (2008)

2008
992
LKB1 and lung cancer: more than the usual suspects.
[18483235] Cancer Res 68(10):3562-5 (2008)

2008
993
mda-9/Syntenin: more than just a simple adapter protein when it comes to cancer metastasis.
[18451132] Cancer Res 68(9):3087-93 (2008)

2008
994
Crucial role of interleukin-4 in the survival of colon cancer stem cells.
[18519657] Cancer Res 68(11):4022-5 (2008)

2008
995
Is tumor growth sustained by rare cancer stem cells or dominant clones?
[18519656] Cancer Res 68(11):4018-21 (2008)

2005
996
Bisphosphonates and cancer-induced bone disease: beyond their antiresorptive activity.
[15958534] Cancer Res 65(12):4971-4 (2005)

2005
997
Tumor dormancy and MYC inactivation: pushing cancer to the brink of normalcy.
[15930260] Cancer Res 65(11):4471-4 (2005)

2009
998
Astrocyte elevated gene-1: far more than just a gene regulated in astrocytes.
[19903854] Cancer Res 69(22):8529-35 (2009)

2009
999
Cell fusion as a hidden force in tumor progression.
[19887616] Cancer Res 69(22):8536-9 (2009)

2009
1000
The role of Myc-induced protein synthesis in cancer.
[19934336] Cancer Res 69(23):8839-43 (2009)

2009
1001
Hijacking the chromatin remodeling machinery: impact of SWI/SNF perturbations in cancer.
[19843852] Cancer Res 69(21):8223-30 (2009)

2009
1002
Development and cancer: at the crossroads of Nodal and Notch signaling.
[19738053] Cancer Res 69(18):7131-4 (2009)

2009
1003
Epithelial-mesenchymal transition and cell cooperativity in metastasis.
[19738043] Cancer Res 69(18):7135-9 (2009)

2009
1004
Acting locally and globally: Myc's ever-expanding roles on chromatin.
[19773445] Cancer Res 69(19):7487-90 (2009)

2009   **Regulatory myeloid suppressor cells in health and disease.**
1005   [19752086] Cancer Res 69(19):7503-6 (2009)

2009   **The transcriptional corepressor CtBP: a foe of multiple tumor suppressors.**
1006   [19155295] Cancer Res 69(3):731-4 (2009)

2006   **The primary cilium in cell signaling and cancer.**
1007   [16818613] Cancer Res 66(13):6463-7 (2006)

2008   **Targeting the eukaryotic translation initiation factor 4E for cancer therapy.**
1008   [18245460] Cancer Res 68(3):631-4 (2008)

2002   **How to calculate the dose of chemotherapy.**
1009   [11953888] Br J Cancer 86(8):1297-302 (2002)

2004   **Targeting the mammalian target of rapamycin (mTOR): a new approach to treating cancer.**
1010   [15365568] Br J Cancer 91(8):1420-4 (2004)

2005   **Role of survivin and its splice variants in tumorigenesis.**
1011   [15611788] Br J Cancer 92(2):212-6 (2005)

2003   **Tissue-selective therapy of cancer.**
1012   [14520435] Br J Cancer 89(7):1147-51 (2003)

2010   **TNF-alpha/NF-kappaB/Snail pathway in cancer cell migration and invasion.**
1013   [20087353] Br J Cancer 102(4):639-44 (2010)

2007   **Gene expression profiling for the diagnosis of acute leukaemia.**
1014   [17146476] Br J Cancer 96(4):535-40 (2007)

2007   **Stem cells of ependymoma.**
1015   [17179988] Br J Cancer 96(1):6-10 (2007)

2007   **ASPP: a new family of oncogenes and tumour suppressor genes.**
1016   [17211478] Br J Cancer 96(2):196-200 (2007)

2009   **The context and potential of epigenetics in oncology.**
1017   [19223907] Br J Cancer 100(4):571-7 (2009)

2009   **Targeting HSP90 for cancer therapy.**
1018   [19401686] Br J Cancer 100(10):1523-9 (2009)

2009   **De novo fatty-acid synthesis and related pathways as molecular targets for cancer therapy.**
1019   [19352381] Br J Cancer 100(9):1369-72 (2009)

2009   **T-regulatory cell modulation: the future of cancer immunotherapy?**
1020   [19384299] Br J Cancer 100(11):1697-703 (2009)

2009   **Molecular classification of solid tumours: towards pathway-driven therapeutics.**
1021   [19367275] Br J Cancer 100(10):1517-22 (2009)

2009   **The state of the art: immune-mediated mechanisms of monoclonal antibodies in cancer therapy.**
1022   [19809433] Br J Cancer 101(11):1807-12 (2009)

2009   **Concepts of epigenetics in prostate cancer development.**
1023   [19002169] Br J Cancer 100(2):240-5 (2009)

2008   **Nf2/Merlin: a coordinator of receptor signalling and intercellular contact.**
1024   [17971776] Br J Cancer 98(2):256-62 (2008)

2005   Small RNAs: classification, biogenesis, and function.
1025   [15750334] Mol Cells 19(1):1-15 (2005)

2007   The present status of cell tracking methods in animal models using magnetic resonance imaging
1026   technology.
      [17464188] Mol Cells 23(2):132-7 (2007)

2009   Reconstitution of chromatoid body-like particles in cultured cells: a novel approach to elucidate the
1027   mechanism of assembly and function of the chromatoid body.
      [19229140] RNA Biol 6(2):165-8 (2009)

2009   Regulation of imprinted expression by macro non-coding RNAs.
1028   [19229135] RNA Biol 6(2):100-6 (2009)

2009   Translation regulation of mRNAs by the fragile X family of proteins through the microRNA pathway.
1029   [19276651] RNA Biol 6(2):175-8 (2009)

2009   Whole genome transcriptome analysis.
1030   [19875928] RNA Biol 6(2):107-12 (2009)

2006   Nailfold capillaroscopy is useful for the diagnosis and follow-up of autoimmune rheumatic diseases.
1031   A future tool for the analysis of microvascular heart involvement?
      [16980724] Rheumatology (Oxford) 45 Suppl 4(-):iv43-6 (2006)

2008   Heberden's nodes and what Heberden could not see: the pivotal role of ligaments in the
1032   pathogenesis of early nodal osteoarthritis and beyond.
      [18390583] Rheumatology (Oxford) 47(9):1278-85 (2008)

2008   Neuropsychiatric lupus and reversible posterior leucoencephalopathy syndrome: a challenging
1033   clinical dilemma.
      [18084001] Rheumatology (Oxford) 47(3):256-62 (2008)

2008   Autoinflammatory diseases: an update of clinical and genetic aspects.
1034   [18388145] Rheumatology (Oxford) 47(7):946-51 (2008)

2008   Germinal centre-like structures in Wegener's granuloma: the morphological basis for autoimmunity?
1035   [18515866] Rheumatology (Oxford) 47(8):1111-3 (2008)

2002   Practice guidelines for tumor marker use in the clinic.
1036   [12142367] Clin Chem 48(8):1151-9 (2002)

2010   A critique of the hypothesis, and a defense of the question, as a framework for experimentation.
1037   [20511448] Clin Chem 56(7):1080-5 (2010)

2010   Peptide lost and found: internal standards and the mass spectrometric quantification of peptides.
1038   [20739635] Clin Chem 56(10):1515-7 (2010)

2010   National Academy of Clinical Biochemistry Laboratory Medicine Practice Guidelines for use of tumor
1039   markers in liver, bladder, cervical, and gastric cancers.
      [20207771] Clin Chem 56(6):e1-48 (2010)

2004   D-dimer testing for deep venous thrombosis: a metaanalysis.
1040   [15142977] Clin Chem 50(7):1136-47 (2004)

2010   Identification of pathogens by mass spectrometry.
1041   [20167691] Clin Chem 56(4):525-36 (2010)

2010   The clinical plasma proteome: a survey of clinical assays for proteins in plasma and serum.
1042   [19884488] Clin Chem 56(2):177-85 (2010)

2007   National Academy of Clinical Biochemistry laboratory medicine practice guidelines: use of cardiac
1043   troponin and B-type natriuretic peptide or N-terminal proB-type natriuretic peptide for etiologies
      other than acute coronary syndromes and heart failure.

[17954494] Clin Chem 53(12):2086-96 (2007)

2007 1044	**Applications of nanobiotechnology in clinical diagnostics.** [17890442] Clin Chem 53(11):2002-9 (2007)

2009
1045
Next-generation sequencing: from basic research to diagnostics.
[19246620] Clin Chem 55(4):641-58 (2009)

2009
1046
National academy of clinical biochemistry laboratory medicine practice guidelines: follow-up testing for metabolic disease identified by expanded newborn screening using tandem mass spectrometry; executive summary.
[19574465] Clin Chem 55(9):1615-26 (2009)

2009
1047
Current issues in measurement and reporting of urinary albumin excretion.
[19028824] Clin Chem 55(1):24-38 (2009)

2006
1048
The MALDI-TOF mass spectrometric view of the plasma proteome and peptidome.
[16644871] Clin Chem 52(7):1223-37 (2006)

2008
1049
Noninvasive optical, electrical, and acoustic methods of total hemoglobin determination.
[18070818] Clin Chem 54(2):264-72 (2008)

2011
1050
Targeting Forkhead box O1 from the concept to metabolic diseases: lessons from mouse models.
[20615072] Antioxid Redox Signal 14(4):649-61 (2011)

2011
1051
Critical role of the nitric oxide/reactive oxygen species balance in endothelial progenitor dysfunction.
[20712407] Antioxid Redox Signal 15(4):933-48 (2011)

2010
1052
Interactions of multiple gas-transducing systems: hallmarks and uncertainties of CO, NO, and H2S gas biology.
[19939208] Antioxid Redox Signal 13(2):157-92 (2010)

2010
1053
Generation and biological activities of oxidized phospholipids.
[19686040] Antioxid Redox Signal 12(8):1009-59 (2010)

2010
1054
Cell signaling by protein carbonylation and decarbonylation.
[19686045] Antioxid Redox Signal 12(3):393-404 (2010)

2010
1055
Oxidative stress and vascular smooth muscle cell growth: a mechanistic linkage by cyclophilin A.
[19747062] Antioxid Redox Signal 12(5):675-82 (2010)

2010
1056
The physics of oxygen delivery: facts and controversies.
[19757988] Antioxid Redox Signal 12(6):683-91 (2010)

2010
1057
Novel insights into hydrogen sulfide--mediated cytoprotection.
[19769484] Antioxid Redox Signal 12(10):1203-17 (2010)

2008
1058
Redox regulation of cell survival.
[18522489] Antioxid Redox Signal 10(8):1343-74 (2008)

2009
1059
Redox-directed cancer therapeutics: molecular mechanisms and opportunities.
[19496700] Antioxid Redox Signal 11(12):3013-69 (2009)

2009
1060
Redox control of the cell cycle in health and disease.
[19505186] Antioxid Redox Signal 11(12):2985-3011 (2009)

2003
1061
Catalysis of protein folding by protein disulfide isomerase and small-molecule mimics.
[13678529] Antioxid Redox Signal 5(4):413-24 (2003)

2008   Molecular mechanisms and clinical implications of reversible protein S-glutathionylation.
1062   [18774901] Antioxid Redox Signal 10(11):1941-88 (2008)

2008   Oxidative stress in Fanconi anemia hematopoiesis and disease progression.
1063   [18627348] Antioxid Redox Signal 10(11):1909-21 (2008)

2010   Heme degradation and vascular injury.
1064   [19697995] Antioxid Redox Signal 12(2):233-48 (2010)

2010   Oxidative protein folding and the Quiescin-sulfhydryl oxidase family of flavoproteins.
1065   [20136510] Antioxid Redox Signal 13(8):1217-30 (2010)

2011   Heme oxygenase in the regulation of vascular biology: from molecular mechanisms to therapeutic opportunities.
1066   [20624029] Antioxid Redox Signal 14(1):137-67 (2011)

2007   Heme oxygenase-1 in tumors: is it a false friend?
1067   [17822372] Antioxid Redox Signal 9(12):2099-117 (2007)

2009   Transcriptional regulatory functions of mammalian AP-endonuclease (APE1/Ref-1), an essential multifunctional protein.
1068   [18715144] Antioxid Redox Signal 11(3):621-38 (2009)

2009   Nitric oxide in health and disease of the nervous system.
1069   [18715148] Antioxid Redox Signal 11(3):541-54 (2009)

2009   The Nrf2/ARE pathway as a potential therapeutic target in neurodegenerative disease.
1070   [18717629] Antioxid Redox Signal 11(3):497-508 (2009)

2009   Catalytic antioxidants and neurodegeneration.
1071   [18754709] Antioxid Redox Signal 11(3):555-70 (2009)

2009   Oxidative stress and autophagy in the regulation of lysosome-dependent neuron death.
1072   [18764739] Antioxid Redox Signal 11(3):481-96 (2009)

2009   Connexins in vascular physiology and pathology.
1073   [18834327] Antioxid Redox Signal 11(2):267-82 (2009)

2009   Mitochondrial reactive oxygen species production in excitable cells: modulators of mitochondrial and cell function.
1074   [19187004] Antioxid Redox Signal 11(6):1373-414 (2009)

2009   NADPH oxidase-dependent signaling in endothelial cells: role in physiology and pathophysiology.
1075   [18783313] Antioxid Redox Signal 11(4):791-810 (2009)

2009   Regulation of NADPH oxidase in vascular endothelium: the role of phospholipases, protein kinases, and cytoskeletal proteins.
1076   [18828698] Antioxid Redox Signal 11(4):841-60 (2009)

2009   Thiol-based redox switches in eukaryotic proteins.
1077   [18999917] Antioxid Redox Signal 11(5):997-1014 (2009)

2009   Iron-based redox switches in biology.
1078   [19021503] Antioxid Redox Signal 11(5):1029-46 (2009)

2009   Mechanistic and kinetic details of catalysis of thiol-disulfide exchange by glutaredoxins and potential mechanisms of regulation.
1079   [19119916] Antioxid Redox Signal 11(5):1059-81 (2009)

2009   Compartmentalization of redox signaling through NADPH oxidase-derived ROS.
1080   [18999986] Antioxid Redox Signal 11(6):1289-99 (2009)

2009
1081

PPARs and the cardiovascular system.
[19061437] Antioxid Redox Signal 11(6):1415-52 (2009)

2009
1082

Redox signaling across cell membranes.
[19061438] Antioxid Redox Signal 11(6):1349-56 (2009)

2009
1083

Lipid rafts and caveolae and their role in compartmentation of redox signaling.
[19061440] Antioxid Redox Signal 11(6):1357-72 (2009)

2009
1084

Vesicle formation and endocytosis: function, machinery, mechanisms, and modeling.
[19113823] Antioxid Redox Signal 11(6):1301-12 (2009)

2009
1085

Electrophysiology of reactive oxygen production in signaling endosomes.
[19207039] Antioxid Redox Signal 11(6):1335-47 (2009)

2005
1086

Role of poly(ADP-ribose) polymerase-1 activation in the pathogenesis of diabetic complications: endothelial dysfunction, as a common underlying theme.
[16356120] Antioxid Redox Signal 7(11-12):1568-80 (2005)

2008
1087

Evolution of catalases from bacteria to humans.
[18498226] Antioxid Redox Signal 10(9):1527-48 (2008)

2008
1088

Thiol chemistry in peroxidase catalysis and redox signaling.
[18479206] Antioxid Redox Signal 10(9):1549-64 (2008)

2008
1089

Intracellular iron transport and storage: from molecular mechanisms to health implications.
[18327971] Antioxid Redox Signal 10(6):997-1030 (2008)

2008
1090

Oxidant and redox signaling in vascular oxygen sensing: implications for systemic and pulmonary hypertension.
[18315496] Antioxid Redox Signal 10(6):1137-52 (2008)

2009
1091

Redox regulation of cell survival by the thioredoxin superfamily: an implication of redox gene therapy in the heart.
[19583492] Antioxid Redox Signal 11(11):2741-58 (2009)

2009
1092

Mitochondrial glutathione, a key survival antioxidant.
[19558212] Antioxid Redox Signal 11(11):2685-700 (2009)

2009
1093

Targeting and regulation of reactive oxygen species generation by Nox family NADPH oxidases.
[19438290] Antioxid Redox Signal 11(10):2607-19 (2009)

2009
1094

NADPH oxidases: molecular understanding finally reaching the clinical level?
[19358633] Antioxid Redox Signal 11(10):2365-70 (2009)

2009
1095

Emerging evidence for the importance of phosphorylation in the regulation of NADPH oxidases.
[19358632] Antioxid Redox Signal 11(10):2429-41 (2009)

2009
1096

Downstream targets and intracellular compartmentalization in Nox signaling.
[19309256] Antioxid Redox Signal 11(10):2467-80 (2009)

2011
1097

The resurgence of niacin: from nicotinic acid to niaspan/laropiprant.
[21809737] Isr Med Assoc J 13(6):368-74 (2011)

2011
1098

Periprocedural complication rate of carotid endarterectomy versus carotid angioplasty and stenting: a retrospective study and review of the literature.
[22097228] Isr Med Assoc J 13(10):601-4 (2011)

2010
1099

Novel multitargeted anticancer oral therapies: sunitinib and sorafenib as a paradigm.
[21090521] Isr Med Assoc J 12(10):628-32 (2010)

2010
1100

Transjugular intrahepatic portosystemic shunt: current indications, patient selection and results.
[21243870] Isr Med Assoc J 12(11):687-91 (2010)

2004
1101

Clinical and laboratory assays in the diagnosis of cutaneous adverse drug reactions.
[14740511] Isr Med Assoc J 6(1):50-1 (2004)

2008
1102

Hereditary angioedema: new hopes for an orphan disease.
[19160940] Isr Med Assoc J 10(12):850-5 (2008)

2009
1103

Pediatric tissue expansion: our experience with 103 expanded flap reconstructive procedures in 41 children.
[19891235] Isr Med Assoc J 11(8):474-9 (2009)

2008
1104

Prediction of neurological diseases by using autoantibodies: wishful thinking come true.
[18300567] Isr Med Assoc J 10(1):29-31 (2008)

2008
1105

The mosaic of autoimmunity: prediction, autoantibodies, and therapy in autoimmune diseases--2008.
[18300564] Isr Med Assoc J 10(1):13-9 (2008)

2008
1106

The mosaic of autoimmunity: hormonal and environmental factors involved in autoimmune diseases--2008.
[18300563] Isr Med Assoc J 10(1):8-12 (2008)

2008
1107

The mosaic of autoimmunity: genetic factors involved in autoimmune diseases--2008.
[18300562] Isr Med Assoc J 10(1):3-7 (2008)

2008
1108

Non-invasive monitoring of inflammation in asthma using exhaled nitric oxide.
[18432031] Isr Med Assoc J 10(2):146-8 (2008)

2005
1109

Fatal traumatic heart wounds: review of 160 autopsy cases.
[16106774] Isr Med Assoc J 7(8):498-501 (2005)

2009
1110

Cerebral venous sinus thrombosis.
[20108557] Isr Med Assoc J 11(11):685-8 (2009)

2006
1111

Cell-penetrating peptides and antimicrobial peptides: how different are they?
[16956326] Biochem J 399(1):1-7 (2006)

2002
1112

Carnitine biosynthesis in mammals.
[11802770] Biochem J 361(Pt 3):417-29 (2002)

2011
1113

Assessing mitochondrial dysfunction in cells.
[21726199] Biochem J 435(2):297-312 (2011)

2011
1114

E2s: structurally economical and functionally replete.
[21158740] Biochem J 433(1):31-42 (2011)

2011
1115

Regulation of cellular iron metabolism.
[21348856] Biochem J 434(3):365-81 (2011)

2011
1116

Diverse mechanisms for activation of Wnt signalling in the ovarian tumour microenvironment.
[21668411] Biochem J 437(1):1-12 (2011)

2010
1117

'Unknown' proteins and 'orphan' enzymes: the missing half of the engineering parts list--and how to find it.
[20001958] Biochem J 425(1):1-11 (2010)

2010
1118

Regulation of mRNA cap methylation.
[20025612] Biochem J 425(2):295-302 (2010)

2003
1119
Deglycosylation of glycoproteins with trifluoromethanesulphonic acid: elucidation of molecular structure and function.
[12974674] Biochem J 376(Pt 2):339-50 (2003)

2003
1120
Regulation and organization of adenylyl cyclases and cAMP.
[12940771] Biochem J 375(Pt 3):517-29 (2003)

2003
1121
A perspective of polyamine metabolism.
[13678416] Biochem J 376(Pt 1):1-14 (2003)

2003
1122
The unique features of glycolytic pathways in Archaea.
[12921536] Biochem J 375(Pt 2):231-46 (2003)

2003
1123
Mammalian molybdo-flavoenzymes, an expanding family of proteins: structure, genetics, regulation, function and pathophysiology.
[12578558] Biochem J 372(Pt 1):15-32 (2003)

2009
1124
AMPK and the biochemistry of exercise: implications for human health and disease.
[19196246] Biochem J 418(2):261-75 (2009)

2009
1125
Connexin43 phosphorylation: structural changes and biological effects.
[19309313] Biochem J 419(2):261-72 (2009)

2008
1126
Ca2+ signalling: a new route to NAADP.
[18333834] Biochem J 411(1):e1-3 (2008)

2008
1127
The TSC1-TSC2 complex: a molecular switchboard controlling cell growth.
[18466115] Biochem J 412(2):179-90 (2008)

2006
1128
Video assisted thoracic surgery in the management of spontaneous pneumothorax: the current status.
[16517799] Postgrad Med J 82(965):179-85 (2006)

2006
1129
Ventilator associated pneumonia.
[16517798] Postgrad Med J 82(965):172-8 (2006)

2011
1130
Republished review: Gene therapy for ocular diseases.
[21705775] Postgrad Med J 87(1029):487-95 (2011)

2005
1131
Important cutaneous manifestations of inflammatory bowel disease.
[16143688] Postgrad Med J 81(959):580-5 (2005)

2004
1132
Intravenous therapy.
[14760169] Postgrad Med J 80(939):1-6 (2004)

2004
1133
Iliopsoas abscesses.
[15299155] Postgrad Med J 80(946):459-62 (2004)

2004
1134
Scabies: more than just an irritation.
[15254301] Postgrad Med J 80(945):382-7 (2004)

2004
1135
An approach to drug induced delirium in the elderly.
[15254302] Postgrad Med J 80(945):388-93 (2004)

2004
1136
Management of haematemesis and melaena.
[15254304] Postgrad Med J 80(945):399-404 (2004)

2004
1137
Gene therapy in clinical medicine.
[15466989] Postgrad Med J 80(948):560-70 (2004)

2003   **Serous effusions: diagnosis of malignancy beyond cytomorphology. An analytic review.**
1138   [14612599] Postgrad Med J 79(936):569-74 (2003)

2003   **Breathlessness in hospitalised adult patients.**
1139   [14707242] Postgrad Med J 79(938):681-5 (2003)

2003   **Assessment and management of pain in infants.**
1140   [12954954] Postgrad Med J 79(934):438-43 (2003)

2003   **Acute glomerulonephritis.**
1141   [12743337] Postgrad Med J 79(930):206-13; quiz 212-3 (2003)

2003   **Evaluation of abnormal liver function tests.**
1142   [12840117] Postgrad Med J 79(932):307-12 (2003)

2003   **What is osteoporosis?**
1143   [12697910] Postgrad Med J 79(929):133-8 (2003)

2007   **Endoscopic mucosal resection of Barrett's oesophagus containing dysplasia or intramucosal cancer.**
1144   [17551066] Postgrad Med J 83(980):367-72 (2007)

2007   **Spontaneous bacterial peritonitis.**
1145   [17551068] Postgrad Med J 83(980):379-83 (2007)

2007   **Management of end stage cardiac failure.**
1146   [17551071] Postgrad Med J 83(980):395-401 (2007)

2007   **Larval therapy from antiquity to the present day: mechanisms of action, clinical applications and future potential.**
1147   [17551073] Postgrad Med J 83(980):409-13 (2007)

2007   **The role of the Intra-aortic balloon pump in supporting children with acute cardiac failure.**
1148   [17488858] Postgrad Med J 83(979):308-11 (2007)

2007   **Forget me not: palliative care for people with dementia.**
1149   [17551065] Postgrad Med J 83(980):362-6 (2007)

2007   **Pneumothorax: an update.**
1150   [17621614] Postgrad Med J 83(981):461-5 (2007)

2007   **Delirium in advanced disease.**
1151   [17675545] Postgrad Med J 83(982):525-8 (2007)

2007   **Bone hydatid disease.**
1152   [17675547] Postgrad Med J 83(982):536-42 (2007)

2007   **Heparin induced thrombocytopenia: diagnosis and management update.**
1153   [17823223] Postgrad Med J 83(983):575-82 (2007)

2007   **Survey of the use of epinephrine (adrenaline) for anaphylaxis by junior hospital doctors.**
1154   [17823230] Postgrad Med J 83(983):610-1 (2007)

2007   **Liver disease in erythropoietic protoporphyria: insights and implications for management.**
1155   [18057171] Postgrad Med J 83(986):739-48 (2007)

2007   **Cardiopulmonary exercise testing and its application.**
1156   [17989266] Postgrad Med J 83(985):675-82 (2007)

2007   **Role of transcranial Doppler ultrasonography in stroke.**
1157   [17989267] Postgrad Med J 83(985):683-9 (2007)

2007 **Psoriasis: advances in pathophysiology and management.**
1158 [17989268] Postgrad Med J 83(985):690-7 (2007)

2007 **Multidetector computed tomographic angiography of the cardiovascular system.**
1159 [17989269] Postgrad Med J 83(985):698-704 (2007)

2007 **How do you treat bleeding disorders with desmopressin?**
1160 [17344569] Postgrad Med J 83(977):159-63 (2007)

2007 **The use of elearning in medical education: a review of the current situation.**
1161 [17403945] Postgrad Med J 83(978):212-6 (2007)

2007 **Management of paraproteinaemia.**
1162 [17403946] Postgrad Med J 83(978):217-23 (2007)

2007 **Classical diseases revisited: transient global amnesia.**
1163 [17403949] Postgrad Med J 83(978):236-9 (2007)

2007 **Cryoglobulinaemic vasculitis: classification and clinical and therapeutic aspects.**
1164 [17308210] Postgrad Med J 83(976):87-94 (2007)

2007 **Understanding frailty.**
1165 [17267673] Postgrad Med J 83(975):16-20 (2007)

2005 **Acute poisoning: understanding 90% of cases in a nutshell.**
1166 [15811881] Postgrad Med J 81(954):204-16 (2005)

2006 **Management of acute ventilatory failure.**
1167 [16822920] Postgrad Med J 82(969):438-45 (2006)

2006 **Diagnostic approach to patients with suspected vasculitis.**
1168 [16891436] Postgrad Med J 82(970):483-8 (2006)

2010 **Advances in diagnostic bronchoscopy.**
1169 [20378726] Am J Respir Crit Care Med 182(5):589-97 (2010)

2010 **Chronic critical illness.**
1170 [20448093] Am J Respir Crit Care Med 182(4):446-54 (2010)

2002 **Ventilator-associated pneumonia.**
1171 [11934711] Am J Respir Crit Care Med 165(7):867-903 (2002)

2004 **Permanent pacemakers and implantable defibrillators: considerations for intensivists.**
1172 [15297272] Am J Respir Crit Care Med 170(9):933-40 (2004)

2005 **Therapeutic hypercapnia: careful science, better trials.**
1173 [15640370] Am J Respir Crit Care Med 171(2):96-7 (2005)

2003 **Pathophysiology and management of pulmonary infections in cystic fibrosis.**
1174 [14555458] Am J Respir Crit Care Med 168(8):918-51 (2003)

2003 **Statement on the care of the child with chronic lung disease of infancy and childhood.**
1175 [12888611] Am J Respir Crit Care Med 168(3):356-96 (2003)

2009 **Attenuated P2X7 pore function as a risk factor for virus-induced loss of asthma control.**
1176 [19201928] Am J Respir Crit Care Med 179(4):265-70 (2009)

2010 **Innate immune recognition in infectious and noninfectious diseases of the lung.**
1177 [20167850] Am J Respir Crit Care Med 181(12):1294-309 (2010)

2010   **Diagnostic testing of patients suspected of primary ciliary dyskinesia.**
1178   [19910612] Am J Respir Crit Care Med 181(4):307-14 (2010)

2007   **Cystic fibrosis pulmonary guidelines: chronic medications for maintenance of lung health.**
1179   [17761616] Am J Respir Crit Care Med 176(10):957-69 (2007)

2007   **Lethal and edema toxins in the pathogenesis of Bacillus anthracis septic shock: implications for**
1180   **therapy.**
   [17095744] Am J Respir Crit Care Med 175(3):211-21 (2007)

2007   **Diaphragm muscle fiber dysfunction in chronic obstructive pulmonary disease: toward a**
1181   **pathophysiological concept.**
   [17413128] Am J Respir Crit Care Med 175(12):1233-40 (2007)

2005   **Investigative bronchoprovocation and bronchoscopy in airway diseases.**
1182   [16020805] Am J Respir Crit Care Med 172(7):807-16 (2005)

2005   **Lung transplantation: opportunities for research and clinical advancement.**
1183   [16020804] Am J Respir Crit Care Med 172(8):944-55 (2005)

2006   **S-nitrosothiol signaling in respiratory biology.**
1184   [16528016] Am J Respir Crit Care Med 173(11):1186-93 (2006)

2006   **Myofibroblast or smooth muscle: do in vitro systems adequately replicate tissue smooth muscle?**
1185   [16894016] Am J Respir Crit Care Med 174(4):364-5 (2006)

2008   **Rhinoorbitocerebral mucormycosis: a case report and literature review.**
1186   [19047969] Med Oral Patol Oral Cir Bucal 13(12):E792-5 (2008)

2007   **Cerebrospinal fluid rhinorrhoea: diagnosis and management.**
1187   [17767107] Med Oral Patol Oral Cir Bucal 12(5):E397-400 (2007)

2008   **Evidence concerning the medical management of caries.**
1188   [18449118] Med Oral Patol Oral Cir Bucal 13(5):E325-30 (2008)

2007   **Boron neutron capture therapy in cancer: past, present and future.**
1189   [17891250] Arq Bras Endocrinol Metabol 51(5):852-6 (2007)

2007   **Nelson's Syndrome.**
1190   [18209878] Arq Bras Endocrinol Metabol 51(8):1392-6 (2007)

2007   **Pediatric Cushing's syndrome: clinical features, diagnosis, and treatment.**
1191   [18209864] Arq Bras Endocrinol Metabol 51(8):1261-71 (2007)

2009   **Hypothalamic regulation of food intake and clinical therapeutic applications.**
1192   [19466203] Arq Bras Endocrinol Metabol 53(2):120-8 (2009)

2002   **Clinical review: hemodynamic monitoring in the intensive care unit.**
1193   [11940266] Crit Care 6(1):52-9 (2002)

2004   **Acute renal failure - definition, outcome measures, animal models, fluid therapy and information**
1194   **technology needs: the Second International Consensus Conference of the Acute Dialysis Quality**
   Initiative (ADQI) Group.
   [15312219] Crit Care 8(4):R204-12 (2004)

2005   **The cuff-leak test: what are we measuring?**
1195   [15693980] Crit Care 9(1):31-3 (2005)

2003   **Bench-to-bedside review: microvascular and airspace linkage in ventilator-induced lung injury.**
1196   [14624683] Crit Care 7(6):435-44 (2003)

2003
1197
Science review: mechanisms of ventilator-induced injury.
[12793874] Crit Care 7(3):233-41 (2003)

2010
1198
Bench-to-bedside review: The role of beta-lactamases in antibiotic-resistant Gram-negative infections.
[20594363] Crit Care 14(3):224 (2010)

2010
1199
Treatment of hypophosphatemia in the intensive care unit: a review.
[20682049] Crit Care 14(4):R147 (2010)

2010
1200
Clinical review: scoring systems in the critically ill.
[20392287] Crit Care 14(2):207 (2010)

2010
1201
Delta inflation: a bias in the design of randomized controlled trials in critical care medicine.
[20429873] Crit Care 14(2):R77 (2010)

2010
1202
Hypertension may be the most important component of hyperdynamic therapy in cerebral vasospasm.
[20497601] Crit Care 14(3):151 (2010)

2010
1203
Laparostomy: why and when?
[20236460] Crit Care 14(2):216 (2010)

2010
1204
Goal-directed or goal-misdirected - how should we interpret the literature?
[20236472] Crit Care 14(2):129 (2010)

2010
1205
Intensive Care Unit-acquired infection as a side effect of sedation.
[20226064] Crit Care 14(2):R30 (2010)

2007
1206
Clinical review: beyond immediate survival from resuscitation-long-term outcome considerations after cardiac arrest.
[18177512] Crit Care 11(6):235 (2007)

2007
1207
Assessment of gas exchange in lung disease: balancing accuracy against feasibility.
[18226175] Crit Care 11(6):182 (2007)

2007
1208
Single-drug therapy or selective decontamination of the digestive tract as antifungal prophylaxis in critically ill patients: a systematic review.
[18067657] Crit Care 11(6):R126 (2007)

2007
1209
Corticosteroids to prevent postextubation upper airway obstruction: the evidence mounts.
[17705879] Crit Care 11(4):156 (2007)

2007
1210
How to evaluate the microcirculation: report of a round table conference.
[17845716] Crit Care 11(5):R101 (2007)

2009
1211
Clinical review: post-extubation laryngeal edema and extubation failure in critically ill adult patients.
[20017891] Crit Care 13(6):233 (2009)

2008
1212
Restoring normoglycaemia: not so harmless.
[18341709] Crit Care 12(1):116 (2008)

2008
1213
Clinical review: Major consequences of illicit drug consumption.
[18279535] Crit Care 12(1):202 (2008)

2008
1214
Bench-to-bedside review: Candida infections in the intensive care unit.
[18279532] Crit Care 12(1):204 (2008)

2010
1215
New therapeutic approaches to mendelian disorders.
[20818846] N Engl J Med 363(9):852-63 (2010)

2010   **Early-stage Hodgkin's lymphoma.**
1216   [20818856] N Engl J Med 363(7):653-62 (2010)

2006   **Clinical practices. Scabies.**
1217   [16625010] N Engl J Med 354(16):1718-27 (2006)

2006   **Clinical practice. Prevention of meningococcal disease.**
1218   [17021322] N Engl J Med 355(14):1466-73 (2006)

2006   **Shattuck Lecture. Nitric oxide and cyclic GMP in cell signaling and drug development.**
1219   [17093251] N Engl J Med 355(19):2003-11 (2006)

2006   **Clinical practice. Acute bronchitis.**
1220   [17108344] N Engl J Med 355(20):2125-30 (2006)

2011   **Microbial genomics and infectious diseases.**
1221   [21793746] N Engl J Med 365(4):347-57 (2011)

2002   **Clinical practice. Herpes zoster.**
1222   [12151472] N Engl J Med 347(5):340-6 (2002)

2011   **Truly emerging--a new disease caused by a novel virus.**
1223   [21410394] N Engl J Med 364(16):1561-3 (2011)

2011   **Iron-chelating therapy for transfusional iron overload.**
1224   [21226580] N Engl J Med 364(2):146-56 (2011)

2011   **Short-term and long-term health risks of nuclear-power-plant accidents.**
1225   [21506737] N Engl J Med 364(24):2334-41 (2011)

2011   **Videos in clinical medicine. Hand hygiene.**
1226   [21449775] N Engl J Med 364(13):e24 (2011)

2011   **Clinical practice. Care of the adult patient after sexual assault.**
1227   [21879901] N Engl J Med 365(9):834-41 (2011)

2010   **Susceptibility pathways in Fanconi's anemia and breast cancer.**
1228   [20484397] N Engl J Med 362(20):1909-19 (2010)

2010   **Genomic medicine--an updated primer.**
1229   [20505179] N Engl J Med 362(21):2001-11 (2010)

2010   **Clinical aspects of pandemic 2009 influenza A (H1N1) virus infection.**
1230   [20445182] N Engl J Med 362(18):1708-19 (2010)

2005   **Clinical practice. Management of newly diagnosed HIV infection.**
1231   [16236741] N Engl J Med 353(16):1702-10 (2005)

2005   **Neuraminidase inhibitors for influenza.**
1232   [16192481] N Engl J Med 353(13):1363-73 (2005)

2005   **Avian influenza A (H5N1) infection in humans.**
1233   [16192482] N Engl J Med 353(13):1374-85 (2005)

2004   **Turner's syndrome.**
1234   [15371580] N Engl J Med 351(12):1227-38 (2004)

2005   **Clinical practice. Rosacea.**
1235   [15728812] N Engl J Med 352(8):793-803 (2005)

2009　**Molecular origins of cancer: Molecular basis of colorectal cancer.**
1236　[20018966] N Engl J Med 361(25):2449-60 (2009)

2003　**Cardiovascular disease.**
1237　[12840094] N Engl J Med 349(1):60-72 (2003)

2003　**Molecular diagnosis of the hematologic cancers.**
1238　[12724484] N Engl J Med 348(18):1777-85 (2003)

2003　**Shattuck lecture: Diversity of the immune repertoire and immunoregulation.**
1239　[12637612] N Engl J Med 348(11):1017-26 (2003)

2003　**Hereditary colorectal cancer.**
1240　[12621137] N Engl J Med 348(10):919-32 (2003)

2007　**Computed tomography--an increasing source of radiation exposure.**
1241　[18046031] N Engl J Med 357(22):2277-84 (2007)

2007　**Clinical practice. Assessment of patients' competence to consent to treatment.**
1242　[17978292] N Engl J Med 357(18):1834-40 (2007)

2007　**Clinical practice. Diverticulitis.**
1243　[18003962] N Engl J Med 357(20):2057-66 (2007)

2007　**Sarcoidosis.**
1244　[18032765] N Engl J Med 357(21):2153-65 (2007)

2007　**Clinical practice. The incidentally discovered adrenal mass.**
1245　[17287480] N Engl J Med 356(6):601-10 (2007)

2007　**Clinical practice. Concussion.**
1246　[17215534] N Engl J Med 356(2):166-72 (2007)

2005　**The Groningen protocol--euthanasia in severely ill newborns.**
1247　[15758003] N Engl J Med 352(10):959-62 (2005)

2005　**Psoriasis.**
1248　[15872205] N Engl J Med 352(18):1899-912 (2005)

2008　**Acute lower respiratory tract infection.**
1249　[18272895] N Engl J Med 358(7):716-27 (2008)

2008　**The challenge of HIV-1 subtype diversity.**
1250　[18403767] N Engl J Med 358(15):1590-602 (2008)

2008　**Cricothyroidotomy.**
1251　[18768957] N Engl J Med 359(10):1073 (2008)

2008　**Clinical practice. Gastroesophageal reflux disease.**
1252　[18923172] N Engl J Med 359(16):1700-7 (2008)

2005　**Clinical practice. Atopic dermatitis.**
1253　[15930422] N Engl J Med 352(22):2314-24 (2005)

2009　**Clinical practice. Postexposure prophylaxis for HIV infection.**
1254　[19864675] N Engl J Med 361(18):1768-75 (2009)

2010　**The rational use of pituitary stimulation tests.**
1255　[20644702] Dtsch Arztebl Int 107(25):437-43 (2010)

2010	The treatment of anterior dental trauma.
1256	[21904590] Dtsch Arztebl Int 108(34-35):565-70 (2010)

2010	The diagnosis and treatment of acute pulmonary embolism.
1257	[20838451] Dtsch Arztebl Int 107(34-35):589-95 (2010)

2010	The post mortem external examination: determination of the cause and manner of death.
1258	[20830284] Dtsch Arztebl Int 107(33):575-86; quiz 587-8 (2010)

2010	The treatment of patients with HIV.
1259	[20703338] Dtsch Arztebl Int 107(28-29):507-15; quiz 516 (2010)

2011	The treatment of spinal metastases.
1260	[21311714] Dtsch Arztebl Int 108(5):71-9; quiz 80 (2011)

2011	Awareness under general anesthesia.
1261	[21285993] Dtsch Arztebl Int 108(1-2):1-7 (2011)

2011	Neonatal screening for metabolic and endocrine disorders.
1262	[21285998] Dtsch Arztebl Int 108(1-2):11-21; quiz 22 (2011)

2011	Photodermatoses: diagnosis and treatment.
1263	[21442060] Dtsch Arztebl Int 108(9):135-41 (2011)

2011	Central venous port systems as an integral part of chemotherapy.
1264	[21442071] Dtsch Arztebl Int 108(9):147-53; quiz 154 (2011)

2011	Obsessive-compulsive disorder in children and adolescents.
1265	[21475565] Dtsch Arztebl Int 108(11):173-9 (2011)

2011	Central oculomotor disturbances and nystagmus: a window into the brainstem and cerebellum.
1266	[21505601] Dtsch Arztebl Int 108(12):197-204 (2011)

2011	Bariatric surgery.
1267	[21655459] Dtsch Arztebl Int 108(20):341-6 (2011)

2011	Current pacemaker and defibrillator therapy.
1268	[21691561] Dtsch Arztebl Int 108(21):372-9; quiz 380 (2011)

2011	The surgical treatment of sleep-related upper airway obstruction.
1269	[21505609] Dtsch Arztebl Int 108(13):216-21 (2011)

2011	The management of psychiatric emergencies.
1270	[21505610] Dtsch Arztebl Int 108(13):222-30 (2011)

2011	Evidence-based treatment of chronic leg ulcers.
1271	[21547162] Dtsch Arztebl Int 108(14):231-7 (2011)

2011	Amniotic membrane transplantation in the human eye.
1272	[21547164] Dtsch Arztebl Int 108(14):243-8 (2011)

2011	Inherited cardiac arrhythmias: diagnosis, treatment, and prevention.
1273	[21977220] Dtsch Arztebl Int 108(37):623-33; quiz 634 (2011)

2011	Ovarian cancer: diagnosis and treatment.
1274	[22025930] Dtsch Arztebl Int 108(38):635-41 (2011)

2011	Failure to thrive in childhood.
1275	[22025931] Dtsch Arztebl Int 108(38):642-9 (2011)

2011 **The diagnosis and treatment of eating disorders.**
1276 [22114627] Dtsch Arztebl Int 108(40):678-85 (2011)

2011 **Treatment strategies for resistant arterial hypertension.**
1277 [22114648] Dtsch Arztebl Int 108(43):725-31 (2011)

2011 **Standardized prehospital treatment of stroke.**
1278 [21966316] Dtsch Arztebl Int 108(36):585-91 (2011)

2011 **Patient care at the 2010 Love Parade in Duisburg, Germany: clinical experiences.**
1279 [21814525] Dtsch Arztebl Int 108(28-29):483-9 (2011)

2011 **Hormonal contraception--what kind, when, and for whom?**
1280 [21814535] Dtsch Arztebl Int 108(28-29):495-505; quiz 506 (2011)

2011 **Negative-pressure wound therapy: systematic review of randomized controlled trials.**
1281 [21712971] Dtsch Arztebl Int 108(22):381-9 (2011)

2011 **Tumors of the central nervous system in children and adolescents.**
1282 [21712972] Dtsch Arztebl Int 108(22):390-7 (2011)

2011 **Uncomplicated urinary tract infections.**
1283 [21776311] Dtsch Arztebl Int 108(24):415-23 (2011)

2011 **The differential diagnosis of hearing loss.**
1284 [21776317] Dtsch Arztebl Int 108(25):433-43; quiz 444 (2011)

2011 **Hemoglobinopathies: clinical manifestations, diagnosis, and treatment.**
1285 [21886666] Dtsch Arztebl Int 108(31-32):532-40 (2011)

2011 **Cluster headache: clinical features and therapeutic options.**
1286 [21912573] Dtsch Arztebl Int 108(33):543-9 (2011)

2011 **Treatment of tobacco dependence.**
1287 [21912578] Dtsch Arztebl Int 108(33):555-64 (2011)

2010 **The origins of colorectal carcinoma: specific nomenclature for different pathways and precursor
1288** **lesions.**
[21085545] Dtsch Arztebl Int 107(43):760-6 (2010)

2010 **New developments in the diagnosis of dementia.**
1289 [20963198] Dtsch Arztebl Int 107(39):677-83 (2010)

2010 **Lewy body and parkinsonian dementia: common, but often misdiagnosed conditions.**
1290 [20963199] Dtsch Arztebl Int 107(39):684-91 (2010)

2010 **The prevention, diagnosis, and treatment of dyslexia.**
1291 [21046003] Dtsch Arztebl Int 107(41):718-26; quiz 27 (2010)

2010 **Boxing-acute complications and late sequelae: from concussion to dementia.**
1292 [21173899] Dtsch Arztebl Int 107(47):835-9 (2010)

2010 **Intra-abdominal adhesions: definition, origin, significance in surgical practice, and treatment
1293** **options.**
[21116396] Dtsch Arztebl Int 107(44):769-75 (2010)

2010 **The diagnosis of urinary tract infection: a systematic review.**
1294 [20539810] Dtsch Arztebl Int 107(21):361-7 (2010)

| 2010 | Decubitus ulcers: pathophysiology and primary prevention. |
| 1295 | [20539816] Dtsch Arztebl Int 107(21):371-81; quiz 382 (2010) |

| 2010 | Child abuse and neglect: diagnosis and management. |
| 1296 | [20396522] Dtsch Arztebl Int 107(13):231-39; quiz 240 (2010) |

| 2010 | The financing of drug trials by pharmaceutical companies and its consequences. Part 1: a qualitative, systematic review of the literature on possible influences on the findings, protocols, and quality of drug trials. |
| 1297 | [20467553] Dtsch Arztebl Int 107(16):279-85 (2010) |

| 2010 | The financing of drug trials by pharmaceutical companies and its consequences: part 2: a qualitative, systematic review of the literature on possible influences on authorship, access to trial data, and trial registration and publication. |
| 1298 | [20490338] Dtsch Arztebl Int 107(17):295-301 (2010) |

| 2008 | Biopsy of tumors of the musculoskeletal system. |
| 1299 | [19626189] Dtsch Arztebl Int 105(27):492-7 (2008) |

| 2008 | Treatment of depressive disorders. |
| 1300 | [19578410] Dtsch Arztebl Int 105(45):782-92 (2008) |

| 2008 | Reconstructive oral and maxillofacial surgery. |
| 1301 | [19578412] Dtsch Arztebl Int 105(47):815-22 (2008) |

| 2010 | Patient safety and error management: what causes adverse events and how can they be prevented? |
| 1302 | [20204120] Dtsch Arztebl Int 107(6):92-9 (2010) |

| 2009 | Shaken baby syndrome: a common variant of non-accidental head injury in infants. |
| 1303 | [19471629] Dtsch Arztebl Int 106(13):211-7 (2009) |

| 2009 | Ultrasonographic screening for the detection of abdominal aortic aneurysms. |
| 1304 | [19946430] Dtsch Arztebl Int 106(41):657-63 (2009) |

| 2010 | Management of patients with acute hyperkalemia. |
| 1305 | [20855477] CMAJ 182(15):1631-5 (2010) |

| 2002 | Bioethics for clinicians: 28. Protestant bioethics. |
| 1306 | [11868645] CMAJ 166(3):339-43 (2002) |

| 2002 | Nephrology: 2. Evaluation of asymptomatic hematuria and proteinuria in adult primary care. |
| 1307 | [11868646] CMAJ 166(3):348-53 (2002) |

| 2011 | Does my dizzy patient have a stroke? A systematic review of bedside diagnosis in acute vestibular syndrome. |
| 1308 | [21576300] CMAJ 183(9):E571-92 (2011) |

| 2011 | Cardiac resynchronization therapy: a meta-analysis of randomized controlled trials. |
| 1309 | [21282316] CMAJ 183(4):421-9 (2011) |

| 2011 | Unintentional weight loss in older adults. |
| 1310 | [21324857] CMAJ 183(4):443-9 (2011) |

| 2011 | Management of acne. |
| 1311 | [21398228] CMAJ 183(7):E430-5 (2011) |

| 2011 | Use of acid-suppressive drugs and risk of pneumonia: a systematic review and meta-analysis. |
| 1312 | [21173070] CMAJ 183(3):310-9 (2011) |

| 2011 | Clinical practice guidelines for the use of noninvasive positive-pressure ventilation and noninvasive continuous positive airway pressure in the acute care setting. |
| 1313 | |

[21324867] CMAJ 183(3):E195-214 (2011)

2011 **San Francisco Syncope Rule to predict short-term serious outcomes: a systematic review.**
1314 [21948723] CMAJ 183(15):E1116-26 (2011)

2010 **Reducing the pain of childhood vaccination: an evidence-based clinical practice guideline**
1315 **(summary).**
[21098067] CMAJ 182(18):1989-95 (2010)

2010 **Developing and selecting interventions for translating knowledge to action.**
1316 [20026633] CMAJ 182(2):E85-8 (2010)

2003 **Diagnosis and management of anaphylaxis.**
1317 [12925426] CMAJ 169(4):307-11 (2003)

2008 **Guidelines for the management of chronic kidney disease.**
1318 [19015566] CMAJ 179(11):1154-62 (2008)

2010 **Selecting educational interventions for knowledge translation.**
1319 [20048013] CMAJ 182(2):E89-93 (2010)

2010 **Monitoring use of knowledge and evaluating outcomes.**
1320 [20083566] CMAJ 182(2):E94-8 (2010)

2010 **Implement research faster.**
1321 [20142393] CMAJ 182(2):176 (2010)

2010 **Prophylaxis of migraine headache.**
1322 [20159899] CMAJ 182(7):E269-76 (2010)

2010 **Knowledge creation: synthesis, tools and products.**
1323 [19884300] CMAJ 182(2):E68-72 (2010)

2010 **The knowledge-to-action cycle: identifying the gaps.**
1324 [19948812] CMAJ 182(2):E73-7 (2010)

2002 **Fire ants in Australia: a new medical and ecological hazard.**
1325 [12064981] Med J Aust 176(11):518-9 (2002)

2003 **Inclusion of patients in clinical trial analysis: the intention-to-treat principle.**
1326 [14558871] Med J Aust 179(8):438-40 (2003)

2003 **Management of acute adult sexual assault.**
1327 [12603187] Med J Aust 178(5):226-30 (2003)

2006 **1. Diagnosis, treatment and prevention of allergic disease: the basics.**
1328 [16922672] Med J Aust 185(4):228-33 (2006)

2011 **IL-17-expressing cells as a potential therapeutic target for treatment of immunological disorders.**
1329 [21441609] Pharmacol Rep 63(1):30-44 (2011)

2011 **Basic mechanisms of antiepileptic drugs and their pharmacokinetic/pharmacodynamic interactions:**
1330 **an update.**
[21602586] Pharmacol Rep 63(2):271-92 (2011)

2011 **Pharmocoepigenetics: a new approach to predicting individual drug responses and targeting new**
1331 **drugs.**
[21602587] Pharmacol Rep 63(2):293-304 (2011)

2011   **Therapeutic potential of adenosine analogues and conjugates.**
1332   [21857072] Pharmacol Rep 63(3):601-17 (2011)

2010   **Red blood cells (RBCs), epoxyeicosatrienoic acids (EETs) and adenosine triphosphate (ATP).**
1333   [20631410] Pharmacol Rep 62(3):468-74 (2010)

2010   **Regulation of cAMP by phosphodiesterases in erythrocytes.**
1334   [20631411] Pharmacol Rep 62(3):475-82 (2010)

2010   **Transcellular biosynthesis of eicosanoids.**
1335   [20631414] Pharmacol Rep 62(3):503-10 (2010)

2010   **Vane's discovery of the mechanism of action of aspirin changed our understanding of its clinical pharmacology.**
1336   [20631416] Pharmacol Rep 62(3):518-25 (2010)

2010   **Cytochrome P450-dependent metabolism of omega-6 and omega-3 long-chain polyunsaturated fatty acids.**
1337   [20631419] Pharmacol Rep 62(3):536-47 (2010)

2005   **Purinoceptors in renal microvessels: adenosine-activated and cytochrome P450 monooxygenase-derived arachidonate metabolites.**
1338   [16415499] Pharmacol Rep 57 Suppl(-):191-5 (2005)

2005   **Drug-induced myopathies. An overview of the possible mechanisms.**
1339   [15849374] Pharmacol Rep 57(1):23-34 (2005)

2005   **Role of nitric oxide, nitroxidative and oxidative stress in wound healing.**
1340   [16415491] Pharmacol Rep 57 Suppl(-):108-19 (2005)

2005   **Inflammatory lipid mediators in ischemic retinopathy.**
1341   [16415498] Pharmacol Rep 57 Suppl(-):169-90 (2005)

2010   **Immunological aspects of epilepsy.**
1342   [20885000] Pharmacol Rep 62(4):592-607 (2010)

2007   **Anti-inflammatory and side effects of cyclooxygenase inhibitors.**
1343   [17652824] Pharmacol Rep 59(3):247-58 (2007)

2007   **Statins: a new insight into their mechanisms of action and consequent pleiotropic effects.**
1344   [18048949] Pharmacol Rep 59(5):483-99 (2007)

2009   **Third-generation antiepileptic drugs: mechanisms of action, pharmacokinetics and interactions.**
1345   [19443931] Pharmacol Rep 61(2):197-216 (2009)

2009   **Pharmacology of dimethyl sulfoxide in cardiac and CNS damage.**
1346   [19443933] Pharmacol Rep 61(2):225-35 (2009)

2007   **Hormonal supplementation in endocrine dysfunction in critically ill patients.**
1347   [17556792] Pharmacol Rep 59(2):139-49 (2007)

2009   **Nitrate tolerance as a model of vascular dysfunction: roles for mitochondrial aldehyde dehydrogenase and mitochondrial oxidative stress.**
1348   [19307691] Pharmacol Rep 61(1):33-48 (2009)

2009   **Mitochondria and vascular pathology.**
1349   [19307700] Pharmacol Rep 61(1):123-30 (2009)

2007   **Hydrogen sulfide (H2S) - the third gas of interest for pharmacologists.**
1350   [17377202] Pharmacol Rep 59(1):4-24 (2007)

2008
1351
Microparticles are vectors of paradoxical information in vascular cells including the endothelium: role in health and diseases.
[18276988] Pharmacol Rep 60(1):75-84 (2008)

2008
1352
Biliverdin reductase: new features of an old enzyme and its potential therapeutic significance.
[18276984] Pharmacol Rep 60(1):38-48 (2008)

2008
1353
NADPH oxidase-derived reactive oxygen species in the regulation of endothelial phenotype.
[18276982] Pharmacol Rep 60(1):21-8 (2008)

2008
1354
Dual control of vascular tone and remodelling by ATP released from nerves and endothelial cells.
[18276981] Pharmacol Rep 60(1):12-20 (2008)

2008
1355
Prostacyclin among prostanoids.
[18276980] Pharmacol Rep 60(1):3-11 (2008)

2008
1356
Pharmacokinetics and pharmacodynamics of aliskiren, an oral direct renin inhibitor.
[19066408] Pharmacol Rep 60(5):623-31 (2008)

2008
1357
Physiology and pharmacological role of the blood-brain barrier.
[19066407] Pharmacol Rep 60(5):600-22 (2008)

2009
1358
Nicotine dependence - human and animal studies, current pharmacotherapies and future perspectives.
[20081230] Pharmacol Rep 61(6):957-65 (2009)

2011
1359
Recent aspects of vasculitis and future direction.
[21921363] Intern Med 50(18):1869-77 (2011)

2011
1360
Diagnosis of Invasive Fungal Disease Using Serum (1â†' 3)-Î²-D-Glucan: A Bivariate Meta-Analysis.
[22082890] Intern Med 50(22):2783-91 (2011)

2004
1361
Circulating endothelial cells and vasculitis.
[15468962] Intern Med 43(8):660-7 (2004)

2004
1362
Endothelial microparticles and the diagnosis of the vasculitides.
[15645643] Intern Med 43(12):1115-9 (2004)

2004
1363
Regression of liver fibrosis in patients treated by interferon.
[15575231] Intern Med 43(10):887-8 (2004)

2007
1364
Neuro-neutrophilic disease: neuro-BehÃ§et disease and neuro-Sweet disease.
[17301507] Intern Med 46(4):153-4 (2007)

2005
1365
Familial pseudohyperkalemia: a rare syndrome, but diverse genetic heterogeneity.
[16157971] Intern Med 44(8):781-2 (2005)

2011
1366
Intimate partner violence - identification and response in general practice.
[22059211] Aust Fam Physician 40(11):852-6 (2011)

2010
1367
Interstitial lung disease - An approach to diagnosis and management.
[20369109] Aust Fam Physician 39(3):106-10 (2010)

2010
1368
Chronic urticaria--assessment and treatment.
[20369115] Aust Fam Physician 39(3):135-8 (2010)

2010
1369
Assessment of the unwell child.
[20485711] Aust Fam Physician 39(5):270-5 (2010)

2004   **Eating disorders in adolescence. An approach to diagnosis and management.**
1370   [14988957] Aust Fam Physician 33(1-2):27-31 (2004)

2007   **Premenstrual disorders in adolescent females-- integrative management.**
1371   [17676186] Aust Fam Physician 36(8):629-30 (2007)

2007   **The vomiting child--what to do and when to consult.**
1372   [17885698] Aust Fam Physician 36(9):684-7 (2007)

2007   **Nausea and vomiting in adults--a diagnostic approach.**
1373   [17885699] Aust Fam Physician 36(9):688-92 (2007)

2005   **Eczema--practical management issues.**
1374   [15887932] Aust Fam Physician 34(5):319-24 (2005)

2009   **Restless legs syndrome.**
1375   [19458798] Aust Fam Physician 38(5):296-300 (2009)

2005   **Glomerulonephritis--management in general practice.**
1376   [16299623] Aust Fam Physician 34(11):907-13 (2005)

2005   **Management of an acute asthma attack.**
1377   [15999162] Aust Fam Physician 34(7):531-4 (2005)

2005   **Migraine and tension headache--a complementary and alternative medicine approach.**
1378   [16113701] Aust Fam Physician 34(8):647-51 (2005)

2009   **Spider bites - Assessment and management.**
1379   [19893831] Aust Fam Physician 38(11):862-7 (2009)

2006   **Leg ulcers - causes and management.**
1380   [16820817] Aust Fam Physician 35(7):480-4 (2006)

2010   **Cystic pancreatic lesions: a pictorial review and management approach.**
1381   [20848066] Singapore Med J 51(8):668-75 (2010)

2011   **Drugs in resuscitation: an update.**
1382   [21879219] Singapore Med J 52(8):596-602 (2011)

2011   **Hypersexual features in Huntington's disease.**
1383   [21731984] Singapore Med J 52(6):e131-3 (2011)

2010   **Is utilisation of computed tomography justified in clinical practice? Part I: application in the emergency department.**
1384   [20428740] Singapore Med J 51(3):200-6 (2010)

2007   **Neurogenic fever.**
1385   [17538744] Singapore Med J 48(6):492-4 (2007)

2007   **Nogo A protein neutralisation and motor cortex computer implants: a future hope for spinal cord injury.**
1386   [17538769] Singapore Med J 48(6):596-7 (2007)

2007   **Refractive surgery: the future of perfect vision?**
1387   [17657376] Singapore Med J 48(8):709-18; quiz 719 (2007)

2007   **Biomechanics of road traffic collision injuries: a clinician's perspective.**
1388   [17609836] Singapore Med J 48(7):693-700; quiz 700 (2007)

2007 1389	**Point-of-care blood ketone testing: screening for diabetic ketoacidosis at the emergency department.** [17975686] Singapore Med J 48(11):986-9 (2007)
2007 1390	**Immunosuppressive therapy in lung injury due to paraquat poisoning: a meta-analysis.** [17975689] Singapore Med J 48(11):1000-5 (2007)
2009 1391	**Colonic pseudo-obstruction.** [19352564] Singapore Med J 50(3):237-44 (2009)
2009 1392	**Stevens-Johnson syndrome and toxic epidermal necrolysis: efficacy of intravenous immunoglobulin and a review of treatment options.** [19224081] Singapore Med J 50(1):29-33 (2009)
2008 1393	**Common benign and malignant neoplasms of the skin.** [18204762] Singapore Med J 49(1):6-17; quiz 18 (2008)
2009 1394	**123I-BMIPP fatty acid analogue imaging is a novel diagnostic and prognostic approach following acute myocardial infarction.** [19907882] Singapore Med J 50(10):943-8 (2009)
2006 1395	**The extrahepatic consequences of cirrhosis.** [16915189] MedGenMed 8(1):59 (2006)
2007 1396	**Extraintestinal manifestations of inflammatory bowel disease: focus on the musculoskeletal, dermatologic, and ocular manifestations.** [17435655] MedGenMed 9(1):55 (2007)
2007 1397	**Physicians of the future will use online content at the point-of-care to guide their decisions. The future is now!** [17435613] MedGenMed 9(1):4 (2007)
2008 1398	**Deliberate self-harm (and attempted suicide).** [19445786] Clin Evid (Online) 2008(-):- (2008)
2009 1399	**Leg cramps.** [19445755] Clin Evid (Online) 2009(-):- (2009)
2009 1400	**Head lice.** [19445766] Clin Evid (Online) 2009(-):- (2009)
2005 1401	**Risk of death with atypical antipsychotic drug treatment for dementia: meta-analysis of randomized placebo-controlled trials.** [16234500] JAMA 294(15):1934-43 (2005)
2008 1402	**A 50-year-old woman addicted to heroin: review of treatment of heroin addiction.** [18594026] JAMA 300(3):314-21 (2008)
2003 1403	**Efficacy of postoperative epidural analgesia: a meta-analysis.** [14612482] JAMA 290(18):2455-63 (2003)
2003 1404	**What clinicians should know about the QT interval.** [12709470] JAMA 289(16):2120-7 (2003)
2008 1405	**A 24-year-old woman with intractable seizures: review of surgery for epilepsy.** [18984876] JAMA 300(21):2527-38 (2008)
2007 1406	**Does this patient have dementia?** [17551132] JAMA 297(21):2391-404 (2007)

2009   **Persistent chest pain and no obstructive coronary artery disease.**
1407   [19351944] JAMA 301(14):1468-74 (2009)

2009   **A 70-year-old woman with shingles: review of herpes zoster.**
1408   [19491172] JAMA 302(1):73-80 (2009)

2009   **Evolving health effects of Pneumocystis: one hundred years of progress in diagnosis and treatment.**
1409   [19549975] JAMA 301(24):2578-85 (2009)

   Canadian Cardiovascular Society Consensus Conference recommendations on heart failure update
2007   **2007: Prevention, management during intercurrent illness or acute decompensation, and use of**
1410   **biomarkers.**
   [17245481] Can J Cardiol 23(1):21-45 (2007)

2007   **Optimizing the delivery and use of a new monoclonal antibody in children with congenital heart**
1411   **disease: a successful provincial respiratory syncytial virus prophylaxis program.**
   [17487291] Can J Cardiol 23(6):463-6 (2007)

2005   **Emergency diagnosis of congestive heart failure: impact of signs and symptoms.**
1412   [16239975] Can J Cardiol 21(11):921-4 (2005)

2011   **Arrhythmogenic right ventricular cardiomyopathy/dysplasia.**
1413   [21940295] Hellenic J Cardiol 52(5):452-61 (2011)

2010   **Diagnostic modalities of the most common forms of secondary hypertension.**
1414   [21169184] Hellenic J Cardiol 51(6):518-29 (2010)

2008   **Ischemia modified albumin: is this marker of ischemia ready for prime time use?**
1415   [18935713] Hellenic J Cardiol 49(4):260-6 (2008)

2007   **Resistance to aspirin and clopidogrel: possible mechanisms, laboratory investigation, and clinical**
1416   **significance.**
   [18196658] Hellenic J Cardiol 48(6):352-63 (2007)

2007   **Pulmonary embolism: pathophysiology, diagnosis, treatment.**
1417   [17489347] Hellenic J Cardiol 48(2):94-107 (2007)

2006   **Inflammatory cardiomyopathy.**
1418   [16752524] Hellenic J Cardiol 47(2):54-65 (2006)

2009   **Fontan operation.**
1419   [19329415] Hellenic J Cardiol 50(2):133-41 (2009)

2009   **Non-classical indications for cardiac resynchronization therapy.**
1420   [19465362] Hellenic J Cardiol 50(3):208-15 (2009)

2008   **Beta-blockers in the treatment of hypertension: latest data and opinions.**
1421   [18350781] Hellenic J Cardiol 49(1):37-47 (2008)

2008   **Electrical storm: a new challenge in the age of implantable defibrillators.**
1422   [18459465] Hellenic J Cardiol 49(2):86-91 (2008)

2008   **Interleukin 7-induced lymphoid neogenesis in arthritis: recapitulation of a fetal developmental**
1423   **programme?**
   [18792823] Swiss Med Wkly 138(35-36):500-5 (2008)

2011   **Patterns in the occurrence and development of tumors.**
1424   [21542975] Chin Med J (Engl) 124(7):1097-104 (2011)

2010   **Cholinergic anti-inflammatory pathway: a possible approach to protect against myocardial ischemia**
1425   **reperfusion injury.**

[21034659] Chin Med J (Engl) 123(19):2720-6 (2010)

2010
1426
Retinopathy of prematurity: an epidemic in the making.
[21034609] Chin Med J (Engl) 123(20):2929-37 (2010)

2004
1427
Pulmonary alveolar proteinosis treated with whole-lung lavage utilizing extracorporeal membrane oxygenation: a case report and review of literatures.
[15569500] Chin Med J (Engl) 117(11):1746-9 (2004)

2008
1428
Factors influencing the natural history of HIV-1 infection.
[19187605] Chin Med J (Engl) 121(24):2613-21 (2008)

2010
1429
Narcolepsy: clinical features, co-morbidities & treatment.
[20308759] Indian J Med Res 131(-):338-49 (2010)

2010
1430
Parasomnias: an overview.
[20308758] Indian J Med Res 131(-):333-7 (2010)

2007
1431
Battered bodies & shattered minds: violence against women in Bangladesh.
[18032809] Indian J Med Res 126(4):341-54 (2007)

2007
1432
Biological & physiological aspects of action of insulin-like growth factor peptide family.
[17598937] Indian J Med Res 125(4):511-22 (2007)

2009
1433
Oedematous malnutrition.
[20090122] Indian J Med Res 130(5):651-4 (2009)

2010
1434
European Respiratory Society guidelines for the diagnosis and management of lymphangioleiomyomatosis.
[20044458] Eur Respir J 35(1):14-26 (2010)

2007
1435
Master switches of T-cell activation and differentiation.
[17400879] Eur Respir J 29(4):804-12 (2007)

2005
1436
Drug-susceptibility testing in tuberculosis: methods and reliability of results.
[15738303] Eur Respir J 25(3):564-9 (2005)

2009
1437
Soluble guanylate cyclase stimulators as a potential therapy for PAH: enthusiasm, pragmatism and concern.
[19336588] Eur Respir J 33(4):717-21 (2009)

2009
1438
Nonthrombotic pulmonary embolism.
[19648522] Eur Respir J 34(2):452-74 (2009)

2008
1439
The biology of oxygen.
[18378783] Eur Respir J 31(4):887-90 (2008)

2009
1440
Endocrinological derangements in COPD.
[19797671] Eur Respir J 34(4):975-96 (2009)

2009
1441
Lymphoid follicles in (very) severe COPD: beneficial or harmful?
[19567605] Eur Respir J 34(1):219-30 (2009)

2010
1442
The role of pulmonary embolectomy in the treatment of acute pulmonary embolism: a literature review from 1968 to 2008.
[20547704] Interact Cardiovasc Thorac Surg 11(3):265-70 (2010)

2010
1443
Chest drain insertion is not a harmless procedure--are we doing it safely?
[20864452] Interact Cardiovasc Thorac Surg 11(6):745-8 (2010)

2009   **Mid-term results of surgery for chronic thromboembolic pulmonary hypertension.**
1462   [19608561] Interact Cardiovasc Thorac Surg 9(4):626-9 (2009)

2009   **Should you stand on the left or the right of a patient with dextrocardia who needs coronary surgery?**
1463   [19638356] Interact Cardiovasc Thorac Surg 9(4):698-702 (2009)

2006   **Levosimendan for patients with impaired left ventricular function undergoing cardiac surgery.**
1464   [17670579] Interact Cardiovasc Thorac Surg 5(3):322-6 (2006)

2006   **Pulmonary inflammatory myofibroblastic tumor associated with histoplasmosis.**
1465   [17670634] Interact Cardiovasc Thorac Surg 5(4):514-6 (2006)

2010   **Role of endothelin receptor A and NADPH oxidase in vascular abnormalities.**
1466   [20859547] Vasc Health Risk Manag 6(-):787-94 (2010)

2010   **The utility of troponin measurement to detect myocardial infarction: review of the current findings.**
1467   [20859540] Vasc Health Risk Manag 6(-):691-9 (2010)

2010   **Natriuretic peptides (BNP and NT-proBNP): measurement and relevance in heart failure.**
1468   [20539843] Vasc Health Risk Manag 6(-):411-8 (2010)

2010   **Heart rate control with adrenergic blockade: clinical outcomes in cardiovascular medicine.**
1469   [20539841] Vasc Health Risk Manag 6(-):387-97 (2010)

2011   **Troponin elevation in conditions other than acute coronary syndromes.**
1470   [22102783] Vasc Health Risk Manag 7(-):597-603 (2011)

2011   **The causes, consequences, and treatment of left or right heart failure.**
1471   [21603593] Vasc Health Risk Manag 7(-):237-54 (2011)

2011   **Surgery in current therapy for infective endocarditis.**
1472   [21603594] Vasc Health Risk Manag 7(-):255-63 (2011)

2011   **A current evaluation of the safety of angiotensin receptor blockers and direct renin inhibitors.**
1473   [21633727] Vasc Health Risk Manag 7(-):297-313 (2011)

2010   **Diabetic cardiomyopathy: from the pathophysiology of the cardiac myocytes to current diagnosis and management strategies.**
1474   [21057575] Vasc Health Risk Manag 6(-):883-903 (2010)

2010   **Ticagrelor: an investigational oral antiplatelet treatment for reduction of major adverse cardiac events in patients with acute coronary syndrome.**
1475   [21057581] Vasc Health Risk Manag 6(-):963-77 (2010)

2010   **Prevention of the renarrowing of coronary arteries using drug-eluting stents in the perioperative period: an update.**
1476   [20957131] Vasc Health Risk Manag 6(-):855-67 (2010)

2010   **New class of agents for treatment of hypertension: focus on direct renin inhibition.**
1477   [20957132] Vasc Health Risk Manag 6(-):869-82 (2010)

2010   **Pitavastatin approved for treatment of primary hypercholesterolemia and combined dyslipidemia.**
1478   [21127702] Vasc Health Risk Manag 6(-):997-1005 (2010)

2010   **Inhaled insulin: overview of a novel route of insulin administration.**
1479   [20234779] Vasc Health Risk Manag 6(-):47-58 (2010)

2009   **Review of tenecteplase (TNKase) in the treatment of acute myocardial infarction.**
1480   [19436656] Vasc Health Risk Manag 5(1):249-56 (2009)

2007
1481
Summary of the 2007 European Society of Hypertension (ESH) and European Society of Cardiology (ESC) guidelines for the management of arterial hypertension.
[18200799] Vasc Health Risk Manag 3(6):783-95 (2007)

2007
1482
Review of biphasic insulin aspart in the treatment of type 1 and 2 diabetes.
[18200811] Vasc Health Risk Manag 3(6):919-35 (2007)

2007
1483
Update on stents: recent studies on the TAXUS stent system in small vessels.
[17969378] Vasc Health Risk Manag 3(4):481-90 (2007)

2007
1484
A review of picotamide in the reduction of cardiovascular events in diabetic patients.
[17583179] Vasc Health Risk Manag 3(1):93-8 (2007)

2007
1485
Effect of lipid-lowering and anti-hypertensive drugs on plasma homocysteine levels.
[17583180] Vasc Health Risk Manag 3(1):99-108 (2007)

2007
1486
Enoxaparin injection for the treatment of high-risk patients with non-ST elevation acute coronary syndrome.
[17580732] Vasc Health Risk Manag 3(2):221-8 (2007)

2008
1487
Measurement of endothelial function and its clinical utility for cardiovascular risk.
[18827914] Vasc Health Risk Manag 4(3):647-52 (2008)

2010
1488
Severe paraquat poisoning: clinical and radiological findings in a survivor.
[20835601] J Bras Pneumol 36(4):513-6 (2010)

2006
1489
Cellular and biochemical bases of chronic obstructive pulmonary disease.
[17273614] J Bras Pneumol 32(3):241-8 (2006)

2011
1490
Magnetic resonance imaging of the chest: current and new applications, with an emphasis on pulmonology.
[21537662] J Bras Pneumol 37(2):242-58 (2011)

2011
1491
Myositis-related interstitial lung disease and antisynthetase syndrome.
[21390438] J Bras Pneumol 37(1):100-9 (2011)

2010
1492
Antituberculosis drugs: drug interactions, adverse effects, and use in special situations. Part 1: first-line drugs.
[21085830] J Bras Pneumol 36(5):626-40 (2010)

2010
1493
Antituberculosis drugs: drug interactions, adverse effects, and use in special situations. Part 2: second line drugs.
[21085831] J Bras Pneumol 36(5):641-56 (2010)

2010
1494
Diagnosis and treatment of pulmonary hypertension: an update.
[21225184] J Bras Pneumol 36(6):795-811 (2010)

2009
1495
The role of oxidative stress in COPD: current concepts and perspectives.
[20126926] J Bras Pneumol 35(12):1227-37 (2009)

2009
1496
Chapter 5--Aspergillosis: from diagnosis to treatment.
[20126927] J Bras Pneumol 35(12):1238-44 (2009)

2009
1497
Chapter 6--paracoccidioidomycosis.
[20126928] J Bras Pneumol 35(12):1245-9 (2009)

2010
1498
Chapter 7: zygomycosis.
[20209316] J Bras Pneumol 36(1):134-41 (2010)

2010
1499
Chapter 8: Fungal infections in immunocompromised patients.
[20209317] J Bras Pneumol 36(1):142-7 (2010)

2007   **Transfusion-related acute lung injury.**
1500   [17724541] J Bras Pneumol 33(2):206-12 (2007)

2009   **Pulmonary eosinophilia.**
1501   [19618037] J Bras Pneumol 35(6):561-73 (2009)

2009   **Chronic interstitial lung diseases in children.**
1502   [19750333] J Bras Pneumol 35(8):792-803 (2009)

2008   **High-resolution computed tomography patterns of diffuse interstitial lung disease with clinical and pathological correlation.**
1503   [18982210] J Bras Pneumol 34(9):715-44 (2008)

2008   **Testing pulmonary vasoreactivity.**
1504   [19009218] J Bras Pneumol 34(10):838-44 (2008)

2009   **Chapter 4--histoplasmosis.**
1505   [20011851] J Bras Pneumol 35(11):1145-51 (2009)

2009   **Chapter 3--pulmonary cryptococcosis.**
1506   [20011850] J Bras Pneumol 35(11):1136-44 (2009)

2009   **Nosocomial pneumonia: importance of the oral environment.**
1507   [20011848] J Bras Pneumol 35(11):1116-24 (2009)

2009   **Primary immunodeficiency diseases: relevant aspects for pulmonologists.**
1508   [19918634] J Bras Pneumol 35(10):1008-17 (2009)

2009   **Chapter 2: coccidioidomycosis.**
1509   [19820819] J Bras Pneumol 35(9):920-30 (2009)

2009   **Chapter 1: laboratory diagnosis of pulmonary mycoses.**
1510   [19820818] J Bras Pneumol 35(9):907-19 (2009)

2009   **Viral pneumonia: epidemiological, clinical, pathophysiological and therapeutic aspects.**
1511   [19820817] J Bras Pneumol 35(9):899-906 (2009)

2006   **Pleurodesis: technique and indications.**
1512   [17268735] J Bras Pneumol 32(4):347-56 (2006)

2010   **Microsporidiosis: epidemiology, clinical data and therapy.**
1513   [20702053] Gastroenterol Clin Biol 34(8-9):450-64 (2010)

2008   **The Surgisis AFP anal fistula plug: a new and reasonable alternative for the treatment of anal fistula.**
1514   [18947949] Gastroenterol Clin Biol 32(11):946-8 (2008)

2005   **Digestive smooth muscle mitochondrial myopathy in patients with mitochondrial-neuro-gastro-intestinal encephalomyopathy (MNGIE).**
1515   [16294144] Gastroenterol Clin Biol 29(8-9):773-8 (2005)

2010   **Autoantibodies and liver disease: uses and abuses.**
1516   [20431809] Can J Gastroenterol 24(4):225-31 (2010)

2003   **Resolution of multiple severe nonsteroidal anti-inflammatory drug-induced colonic strictures with prednisone therapy: a case report and review of the literature.**
1517   [12945011] Can J Gastroenterol 17(8):497-500 (2003)

2003   **Lymphocytic and collagenous colitis: the emerging entity of microscopic colitis. An update on pathophysiology, diagnosis and management.**
1518   [12915915] Can J Gastroenterol 17(7):425-32 (2003)

2007
1519
Congenital cholestatic syndromes: what happens when children grow up?
[18026579] Can J Gastroenterol 21(11):743-51 (2007)

2007
1520
Oral manifestations of gastrointestinal diseases.
[17431513] Can J Gastroenterol 21(4):241-4 (2007)

2009
1521
Relevance of segmental colitis with diverticulosis (SCAD) to other forms of inflammatory bowel disease.
[19543576] Can J Gastroenterol 23(6):439-40 (2009)

2005
1522
Extradigestive manifestation of Helicobacter pylori infection in children and adolescents.
[16010304] Can J Gastroenterol 19(7):421-4 (2005)

2002
1523
Blood-brain barrier breakdown in septic encephalopathy and brain tumours.
[12162731] J Anat 200(6):639-46 (2002)

2002
1524
Axons and glial interfaces: ultrastructural studies.
[12090407] J Anat 200(4):415-30 (2002)

2002
1525
Endothelial barriers: from hypothetical pores to membrane proteins.
[12162722] J Anat 200(6):541-8 (2002)

2002
1526
Intracellular signalling involved in modulating human endothelial barrier function.
[12162723] J Anat 200(6):549-60 (2002)

2002
1527
Extracellular matrix, junctional integrity and matrix metalloproteinase interactions in endothelial permeability regulation.
[12162724] J Anat 200(6):561-74 (2002)

2002
1528
Aquaporin water channels and endothelial cell function.
[12162729] J Anat 200(6):617-27 (2002)

2002
1529
Structure, function and evolution of the gas exchangers: comparative perspectives.
[12430953] J Anat 201(4):281-304 (2002)

2002
1530
The structural basis of pulmonary hypertension in chronic lung disease: remodelling, rarefaction or angiogenesis?
[12430958] J Anat 201(4):335-48 (2002)

2004
1531
Lymphatics at the crossroads of angiogenesis and lymphangiogenesis.
[15198686] J Anat 204(6):433-49 (2004)

2004
1532
Ventrally emigrating neural tube (VENT) cells: a second neural tube-derived cell population.
[15291792] J Anat 205(2):79-98 (2004)

2004
1533
Cardiac anatomy revisited.
[15379923] J Anat 205(3):159-77 (2004)

2007
1534
Molecular mechanisms in the formation of the medial longitudinal fascicle.
[17623036] J Anat 211(2):177-87 (2007)

2007
1535
Evolution of the amygdaloid complex in vertebrates, with special reference to the anamnio-amniotic transition.
[17634058] J Anat 211(2):151-63 (2007)

2007
1536
Comparative aspects of cortical neurogenesis in vertebrates.
[17634059] J Anat 211(2):164-76 (2007)

2007
1537
Slit-Robo interactions during cortical development.
[17553100] J Anat 211(2):188-98 (2007)

2007
1538
Contribution of endothelial cells to organogenesis: a modern reappraisal of an old Aristotelian concept.
[17683480] J Anat 211(4):415-27 (2007)

2007
1539
Morphological and physiological interactions of NG2-glia with astrocytes and neurons.
[17459143] J Anat 210(6):661-70 (2007)

2005
1540
The subiculum: what it does, what it might do, and what neuroanatomy has yet to tell us.
[16185252] J Anat 207(3):271-82 (2005)

2005
1541
Deer antlers: a zoological curiosity or the key to understanding organ regeneration in mammals?
[16313394] J Anat 207(5):603-18 (2005)

2005
1542
Neurulation in the cranial region--normal and abnormal.
[16313396] J Anat 207(5):623-35 (2005)

2005
1543
Astrocytes and NG2-glia: what's in a name?
[16367796] J Anat 207(6):687-93 (2005)

2005
1544
Synantocytes: the fifth element.
[16367797] J Anat 207(6):695-706 (2005)

2005
1545
NG2-expressing cells as oligodendrocyte progenitors in the normal and demyelinated adult central nervous system.
[16367798] J Anat 207(6):707-16 (2005)

2005
1546
Evolution of cranial development and the role of neural crest: insights from amphibians.
[16313386] J Anat 207(5):437-46 (2005)

2008
1547
A natural history of the human mind: tracing evolutionary changes in brain and cognition.
[18380864] J Anat 212(4):426-54 (2008)

2008
1548
Hominin life history: reconstruction and evolution.
[18380863] J Anat 212(4):394-425 (2008)

2008
1549
The environmental context of human evolutionary history in Eurasia and Africa.
[18380862] J Anat 212(4):377-93 (2008)

2008
1550
The hominin fossil record: taxa, grades and clades.
[18380861] J Anat 212(4):354-76 (2008)

2007
1551
Intrapartum ultrasound.
[17659656] Ultrasound Obstet Gynecol 30(2):123-39 (2007)

2006
1552
Support vector machines versus logistic regression: improving prospective performance in clinical decision-making.
[16715467] Ultrasound Obstet Gynecol 27(6):607-8 (2006)

2010
1553
Invisible dermatoses.
[20445293] Indian J Dermatol Venereol Leprol 76(3):239-48 (2010)

2010
1554
Lupus band test.
[20445312] Indian J Dermatol Venereol Leprol 76(3):298-300 (2010)

2010
1555
Named bodies in dermatology.
[20228564] Indian J Dermatol Venereol Leprol 76(2):206-12 (2010)

2010
1556
Topical corticosteroid use in children: adverse effects and how to minimize them.
[20445290] Indian J Dermatol Venereol Leprol 76(3):225-8 (2010)

2008   **Pathogenesis, clinical features and pathology of chronic arsenicosis.**
1557   [19171978] Indian J Dermatol Venereol Leprol 74(6):559-70 (2008)

2008   **Arsenicosis: diagnosis and treatment.**
1558   [19171979] Indian J Dermatol Venereol Leprol 74(6):571-81 (2008)

2008   **Epidemiology and prevention of chronic arsenicosis: an Indian perspective.**
1559   [19171980] Indian J Dermatol Venereol Leprol 74(6):582-93 (2008)

2010   **Retapamulin: a novel topical antibiotic.**
1560   [20061745] Indian J Dermatol Venereol Leprol 76(1):77-9 (2010)

2007   **Etiopathogenesis of pruritus due to systemic causes: Implications for treatment.**
1561   [17675726] Indian J Dermatol Venereol Leprol 73(4):215-7 (2007)

2007   **Minimizing side effects of systemic corticosteroids in children.**
1562   [17675727] Indian J Dermatol Venereol Leprol 73(4):218-21 (2007)

2007   **An approach to the diagnosis of neutrophilic dermatoses: A histopathological perspective.**
1563   [17675728] Indian J Dermatol Venereol Leprol 73(4):222-30 (2007)

2007   **Art and science of patch testing.**
1564   [17921606] Indian J Dermatol Venereol Leprol 73(5):289-91 (2007)

2009   **Acne in India: guidelines for management - IAA consensus document.**
1565   [19282578] Indian J Dermatol Venereol Leprol 75 Suppl 1(-):1-62 (2009)

2009   **Sutures and suturing techniques in skin closure.**
1566   [19584482] Indian J Dermatol Venereol Leprol 75(4):425-34 (2009)

2007   **Heart failure surgery: a speciality in itself.**
1567   [17679356] Scand J Surg 96(2):140-53 (2007)

2007   **Ventricular structures must be understood during surgical restoration for heart failure.**
1568   [17679359] Scand J Surg 96(2):164-76 (2007)

2007   **Management of severe sepsis of abdominal origin.**
1569   [17966743] Scand J Surg 96(3):184-96 (2007)

2007   **Intra-abdominal hypertension and the abdominal compartment syndrome.**
1570   [17966744] Scand J Surg 96(3):197-204 (2007)

2007   **Multidisciplinary approach for patients with pelvic fractures and hemodynamic instability.**
1571   [18265853] Scand J Surg 96(4):272-80 (2007)

2007   **Natural course of incisional hernia and indications for repair.**
1572   [18265856] Scand J Surg 96(4):293-6 (2007)

2011   **An essential role for programmed death-1 in the control of autoimmunity: implications for the**
1573   **future of hematopoietic stem cell transplantation.**
       [21823886] Future Oncol 7(8):929-32 (2011)

2010   **Regulation of cancer germline antigen gene expression: implications for cancer immunotherapy.**
1574   [20465387] Future Oncol 6(5):717-32 (2010)

2010   **Lipid rafts, death receptors and CASMERs: new insights for cancer therapy.**
1575   [20373862] Future Oncol 6(4):491-4 (2010)

2010   **AMPK as a metabolic tumor suppressor: control of metabolism and cell growth.**
1576   [20222801] Future Oncol 6(3):457-70 (2010)

2009   **The TGF-beta paradox in human cancer: an update.**
1577   [19284383] Future Oncol 5(2):259-71 (2009)

2008   **PAX5 and B-cell neoplasms: transformation through presentation.**
1578   [18240995] Future Oncol 4(1):5-9 (2008)

2009   **Epithelial-mesenchymal transition in hepatocellular carcinoma.**
1579   [19852728] Future Oncol 5(8):1169-79 (2009)

2009   **Mechanisms of the epithelial-mesenchymal transition by TGF-beta.**
1580   [19852727] Future Oncol 5(8):1145-68 (2009)

2007   **Contrast agents for hepatic MRI.**
1581   [17921081] Cancer Imaging 7 Spec No A(-):S24-7 (2007)

2007   **PET/CT imaging: what radiologists need to know.**
1582   [17921089] Cancer Imaging 7 Spec No A(-):S95-9 (2007)

2009   **Imaging of the unusual pediatric 'blastomas'.**
1583   [19237343] Cancer Imaging 9(-):1-11 (2009)

2005   **Ultrasound of thyroid cancer.**
1584   [16361145] Cancer Imaging 5(-):157-66 (2005)

2002   **Psychoanatomical substrates of BÃ¡lint's syndrome.**
1585   [11796765] J Neurol Neurosurg Psychiatry 72(2):162-78 (2002)

2005   **Interventional neuroradiology.**
1586   [16107390] J Neurol Neurosurg Psychiatry 76 Suppl 3(-):iii48-iii63 (2005)

2005   **The clinical assessment of the patient with early dementia.**
1587   [16291917] J Neurol Neurosurg Psychiatry 76 Suppl 5(-):v15-24 (2005)

2005   **Neuropathological investigation of dementia: a guide for neurologists.**
1588   [16291923] J Neurol Neurosurg Psychiatry 76 Suppl 5(-):v8-14 (2005)

2005   **Present and future drug treatment for Parkinson's disease.**
1589   [16227533] J Neurol Neurosurg Psychiatry 76(11):1472-8 (2005)

2004   **Brain tumours: classification and genes.**
1590   [15146033] J Neurol Neurosurg Psychiatry 75 Suppl 2(-):ii2-11 (2004)

2004   **Pituitary disease: presentation, diagnosis, and management.**
1591   [15316045] J Neurol Neurosurg Psychiatry 75 Suppl 3(-):iii47-52 (2004)

2004   **Neuro-ophthalmology: examination and investigation.**
1592   [15564427] J Neurol Neurosurg Psychiatry 75 Suppl 4(-):iv2-11 (2004)

2007   **Notes on the kidney and its diseases for the neurologist.**
1593   [17435183] J Neurol Neurosurg Psychiatry 78(5):444-9 (2007)

2007   **A review of screening tests for cognitive impairment.**
1594   [17178826] J Neurol Neurosurg Psychiatry 78(8):790-9 (2007)

2007   **Neuroimaging findings in human prion disease.**
1595   [17135459] J Neurol Neurosurg Psychiatry 78(7):664-70 (2007)

2007   **Neurological control of human sexual behaviour: insights from lesion studies.**
1596   [17189299] J Neurol Neurosurg Psychiatry 78(10):1042-9 (2007)

2007   **Clinical diagnosis and misdiagnosis of sleep disorders.**
1597   [18024690] J Neurol Neurosurg Psychiatry 78(12):1293-7 (2007)

2007   **Imaging of vertebral artery stenosis: a systematic review.**
1598   [17287234] J Neurol Neurosurg Psychiatry 78(11):1218-25 (2007)

2005   **Functional symptoms in neurology: management.**
1599   [15718216] J Neurol Neurosurg Psychiatry 76 Suppl 1(-):i13-21 (2005)

2005   **Functional symptoms and signs in neurology: assessment and diagnosis.**
1600   [15718217] J Neurol Neurosurg Psychiatry 76 Suppl 1(-):i2-12 (2005)

2005   **Cognitive assessment for clinicians.**
1601   [15718218] J Neurol Neurosurg Psychiatry 76 Suppl 1(-):i22-30 (2005)

2005   **Neurological syndromes which can be mistaken for psychiatric conditions.**
1602   [15718219] J Neurol Neurosurg Psychiatry 76 Suppl 1(-):i31-38 (2005)

2005   **Recognising and evaluating disordered mental states: a guide for neurologists.**
1603   [15718220] J Neurol Neurosurg Psychiatry 76 Suppl 1(-):i39-44 (2005)

2010   **Progressive multifocal leukoencephalopathy in individuals with minimal or occult immunosuppression.**
1604   [19828476] J Neurol Neurosurg Psychiatry 81(3):247-54 (2010)

2010   **Ringing ears: the neuroscience of tinnitus.**
1605   [21068300] J Neurosci 30(45):14972-9 (2010)

2010   **Cognition enhancement strategies.**
1606   [21068302] J Neurosci 30(45):14987-92 (2010)

2010   **Toward the second generation of optogenetic tools.**
1607   [21068304] J Neurosci 30(45):14998-5004 (2010)

2005   **Do we know what the early visual system does?**
1608   [16291931] J Neurosci 25(46):10577-97 (2005)

2005   **Neurobiological mechanisms of the placebo effect.**
1609   [16280578] J Neurosci 25(45):10390-402 (2005)

2004   **Mechanisms and roles of axon-Schwann cell interactions.**
1610   [15496660] J Neurosci 24(42):9250-60 (2004)

2008   **Inherited neuronal ion channelopathies: new windows on complex neurological diseases.**
1611   [19005038] J Neurosci 28(46):11768-77 (2008)

2008   **Habenula: crossroad between the basal ganglia and the limbic system.**
1612   [19005047] J Neurosci 28(46):11825-9 (2008)

2007   **Biomimetic brain machine interfaces for the control of movement.**
1613   [17978021] J Neurosci 27(44):11842-6 (2007)

2008   **Anxious to drink: gabapentin normalizes GABAergic transmission in the central amygdala and reduces symptoms of ethanol dependence.**
1614   [18784287] J Neurosci 28(37):9087-9 (2008)

2009   **Corticostriatal Interactions during Learning, Memory Processing, and Decision Making.**
1615   [19828796] J Neurosci 29(41):12831-8 (2009)

2009   **Cycling behavior and memory formation.**
1616   [19828795] J Neurosci 29(41):12824-30 (2009)

2009   **Understanding the role of DISC1 in psychiatric disease and during normal development.**
1617   [19828788] J Neurosci 29(41):12768-75 (2009)

2009   **Extrasynaptic GABAA receptors: form, pharmacology, and function.**
1618   [19828786] J Neurosci 29(41):12757-63 (2009)

2004   **Pancreatic pseudocysts in the 21st century. Part I: classification, pathophysiology, anatomic considerations and treatment.**
1619   [14730118] JOP 5(1):8-24 (2004)

2004   **Pancreatic pseudocysts in the 21st century. Part II: natural history.**
1620   [15007187] JOP 5(2):64-70 (2004)

2003   **Preventing post-ERCP pancreatitis: where are we?**
1621   [12555013] JOP 4(1):22-32 (2003)

2008   **Ritonavir and disulfiram may be synergistic in lowering active interleukin-18 levels in acute pancreatitis, and thereby hasten recovery.**
1622   [18469453] JOP 9(3):350-3 (2008)

2011   **Management of von Hippel-Lindau disease-associated CNS lesions.**
1623   [21955200] Expert Rev Neurother 11(10):1433-41 (2011)

2011   **Reversible cerebral vasoconstriction syndrome: current and future perspectives.**
1624   [21864073] Expert Rev Neurother 11(9):1265-76 (2011)

2007   **Dementia syndromes: evaluation and treatment.**
1625   [17425495] Expert Rev Neurother 7(4):407-22 (2007)

2009   **How do stroke units enhance stroke recovery?**
1626   [19344295] Expert Rev Neurother 9(4):431-4 (2009)

2009   **Pain catastrophizing: a critical review.**
1627   [19402782] Expert Rev Neurother 9(5):745-58 (2009)

2008   **Electron microscopy of trypanosomes--a historical view.**
1628   [18660983] Mem Inst Oswaldo Cruz 103(4):313-25 (2008)

2011   **Meeting Report: Mode(s) of Action of Asbestos and Related Mineral Fibers.**
1629   [21807578] Environ Health Perspect 119(12):1806-10 (2011)

2004   **The science and practice of carcinogen identification and evaluation.**
1630   [15345338] Environ Health Perspect 112(13):1269-74 (2004)

2003   **Large effects from small exposures. I. Mechanisms for endocrine-disrupting chemicals with estrogenic activity.**
1631   [12826473] Environ Health Perspect 111(8):994-1006 (2003)

2007   **Endocrine-disrupting potential of bisphenol A, bisphenol A dimethacrylate, 4-n-nonylphenol, and 4-n-octylphenol in vitro: new data and a brief review.**
1632   [18174953] Environ Health Perspect 115 Suppl 1(-):69-76 (2007)

2007   **Hormesis and its place in nonmonotonic dose-response relationships: some scientific reality checks.**
1633   [17450215] Environ Health Perspect 115(4):500-6 (2007)

2005   **Cytoskeleton and cell cycle control during meiotic maturation of the mouse oocyte: integrating time and space.**
1634   [16322540] Reproduction 130(6):801-11 (2005)

2004   **Embryonic diapause and its regulation.**
1635   [15579584] Reproduction 128(6):669-78 (2004)

2008   **Blastocyst elongation, trophoblastic differentiation, and embryonic pattern formation.**
1636   [18239048] Reproduction 135(2):181-95 (2008)

2009   **Current management of human granulocytic anaplasmosis, human monocytic ehrlichiosis and**
1637   **Ehrlichia ewingii ehrlichiosis.**
   [19681699] Expert Rev Anti Infect Ther 7(6):709-22 (2009)

2009   **The vitamin D-antimicrobial peptide pathway and its role in protection against infection.**
1638   [19895218] Future Microbiol 4(9):1151-65 (2009)

2009   **A structural and functional perspective of alphavirus replication and assembly.**
1639   [19722838] Future Microbiol 4(7):837-56 (2009)

2004   **Accounting for historical information in designing experiments: the Bayesian approach.**
1640   [15536267] Ann Ist Super Sanita 40(2):173-9 (2004)

2010   **HIV virology and pathogenetic mechanisms of infection: a brief overview.**
1641   [20348614] Ann Ist Super Sanita 46(1):5-14 (2010)

2010   **Laboratory diagnostics for HIV infection.**
1642   [20348616] Ann Ist Super Sanita 46(1):24-33 (2010)

2010   **Suggested strategies for the laboratory diagnosis of HIV infection in Italy.**
1643   [20348617] Ann Ist Super Sanita 46(1):34-41 (2010)

2010   **Bird populations as sentinels of endocrine disrupting chemicals.**
1644   [20348622] Ann Ist Super Sanita 46(1):81-8 (2010)

2009   **The micronucleus assay in radiation accidents.**
1645   [19861730] Ann Ist Super Sanita 45(3):260-4 (2009)

2010   **Pruritus: control of itch in patients undergoing dialysis.**
1646   [20361169] Skin Therapy Lett 15(2):1-5 (2010)

2007   **Hydromineral neuroendocrinology: mechanism of sensing sodium levels in the mammalian brain.**
1647   [17350991] Exp Physiol 92(3):513-22 (2007)

2011   **Noncompaction cardiomyopathy: a current view.**
1648   [21894393] Arq Bras Cardiol 97(1):e13-9 (2011)

2007   **Mechanisms and treatment of resistant hypertension.**
1649   [17664996] Arq Bras Cardiol 88(6):683-92 (2007)

2008   **Role of autoantibodies in the physiopathology of Chagas' disease.**
1650   [19009179] Arq Bras Cardiol 91(4):257-62, 281-6 (2008)

2010   **The active role of venous congestion in the pathophysiology of acute decompensated heart failure.**
1651   [20089219] Rev Esp Cardiol 63(1):5-8 (2010)

2009   **Brugada syndrome.**
1652   [19889341] Rev Esp Cardiol 62(11):1297-315 (2009)

2006   **Retinal prostheses for the blind.**
1653   [16625261] Ann Acad Med Singapore 35(3):137-44 (2006)

2004   **Using natural STOP growth signals to prevent excessive axial elongation and the development of**
1654   **myopia.**

[15008556] Ann Acad Med Singapore 33(1):16-20 (2004)

2010   **Genome-wide association studies: promises and pitfalls.**
1655   [20237726] Ann Acad Med Singapore 39(2):77-8 (2010)

2011   **Therapy in pneumonia: what is beyond antibiotics?**
1656   [21325697] Neth J Med 69(1):21-6 (2011)

2011   **Type B lactic acidosis in solid malignancies.**
1657   [21444936] Neth J Med 69(3):120-3 (2011)

2009   **Magnetic resonance imaging and spectroscopy methods for molecular imaging.**
1658   [20016450] Q J Nucl Med Mol Imaging 53(6):565-85 (2009)

2007   **Nuclear imaging in cancer theranostics.**
1659   [17420716] Q J Nucl Med Mol Imaging 51(2):152-63 (2007)

2007   **Pitfalls in PET/CT interpretation.**
1660   [17464270] Q J Nucl Med Mol Imaging 51(3):235-43 (2007)

2005   **The present role of nuclear cardiology in clinical practice.**
1661   [15724135] Q J Nucl Med Mol Imaging 49(1):43-58 (2005)

2005   **Assessment of myocardial viability in chronic ischemic heart disease: current status.**
1662   [15724138] Q J Nucl Med Mol Imaging 49(1):81-96 (2005)

2005   **The many ways to myocardial perfusion imaging.**
1663   [15724132] Q J Nucl Med Mol Imaging 49(1):4-18 (2005)

2005   **Gated single-photon emission computed tomography. The present-day "one-stop-shop" for cardiac**
1664   **imaging.**
    [15724133] Q J Nucl Med Mol Imaging 49(1):19-29 (2005)

2009   **Assessing tumor hypoxia by positron emission tomography with Cu-ATSM.**
1665   [19293767] Q J Nucl Med Mol Imaging 53(2):193-200 (2009)

2008   **Oncologic PET tracers beyond [(18)F]FDG and the novel quantitative approaches in PET imaging.**
1666   [18235421] Q J Nucl Med Mol Imaging 52(1):50-65 (2008)

2008   **Radiometal complexes: characterization and relevant in vitro studies.**
1667   [18480740] Q J Nucl Med Mol Imaging 52(3):222-34 (2008)

2008   **In vitro receptor binding assays: general methods and considerations.**
1668   [18475249] Q J Nucl Med Mol Imaging 52(3):245-53 (2008)

2008   **Bifunctional chelates for metal nuclides.**
1669   [18043537] Q J Nucl Med Mol Imaging 52(2):166-73 (2008)

2009   **Recombinant human TSH (rhTSH) in 2009: new perspectives in diagnosis and therapy.**
1670   [19910902] Q J Nucl Med Mol Imaging 53(5):490-502 (2009)

2009   **Potential value of elastosonography in the diagnosis of malignancy in thyroid nodules.**
1671   [19910898] Q J Nucl Med Mol Imaging 53(5):455-64 (2009)

2010   **Vitamin D and the intracrinology of innate immunity.**
1672   [20156523] Mol Cell Endocrinol 321(2):103-11 (2010)

2011   **The anti-inflammatory and immunosuppressive effects of glucocorticoids, recent developments and**
1673   **mechanistic insights.**
    [20398732] Mol Cell Endocrinol 335(1):2-13 (2011)

2009
1674
NADPH oxidases and angiotensin II receptor signaling.
[19059306] Mol Cell Endocrinol 302(2):148-58 (2009)

2009
1675
New genes and/or molecular pathways associated with adrenal hyperplasias and related adrenocortical tumors.
[19063937] Mol Cell Endocrinol 300(1-2):152-7 (2009)

2009
1676
Endocrine disrupters as obesogens.
[19433244] Mol Cell Endocrinol 304(1-2):19-29 (2009)

2009
1677
Effects of bisphenol A on adipokine release from human adipose tissue: Implications for the metabolic syndrome.
[19433247] Mol Cell Endocrinol 304(1-2):49-54 (2009)

2009
1678
Molecular mechanisms regulating glucocorticoid sensitivity and resistance.
[19000736] Mol Cell Endocrinol 300(1-2):7-16 (2009)

2009
1679
The sweeter side of ACE2: physiological evidence for a role in diabetes.
[18948167] Mol Cell Endocrinol 302(2):193-202 (2009)

2010
1680
Hemoptysis in children.
[20371892] Indian Pediatr 47(3):245-54 (2010)

2004
1681
Management of edema in nephrotic syndrome.
[15347866] Indian Pediatr 41(8):787-95 (2004)

2003
1682
Diagnosis and treatment of disseminated intravascular coagulation.
[12951374] Indian Pediatr 40(8):721-30 (2003)

2007
1683
Simple clinical sings to identify severe neonatal illness.
[18057476] Indian Pediatr 44(11):814-6 (2007)

2009
1684
Drug therapy of cardiac diseases in children.
[19383992] Indian Pediatr 46(4):310-38 (2009)

2009
1685
Guidelines for diagnosis and management of childhood epilepsy.
[19717860] Indian Pediatr 46(8):681-98 (2009)

2009
1686
Structural alterations in peptide-MHC recognition by self-reactive T cell receptors.
[19699075] Curr Opin Immunol 21(6):590-5 (2009)

2008
1687
Peripheral B cell subsets.
[18434123] Curr Opin Immunol 20(2):149-57 (2008)

2009
1688
AIRE in the thymus and beyond.
[19833494] Curr Opin Immunol 21(6):582-9 (2009)

2009
1689
Pulmonary alveolar proteinosis, a primary immunodeficiency of impaired GM-CSF stimulation of macrophages.
[19796925] Curr Opin Immunol 21(5):514-21 (2009)

2008
1690
Autophagy and antiviral immunity.
[18262399] Curr Opin Immunol 20(1):23-9 (2008)

2008
1691
Antigen presentation by monocytes and monocyte-derived cells.
[18160272] Curr Opin Immunol 20(1):52-60 (2008)

2008
1692
Do the peptide-binding properties of diabetogenic class II molecules explain autoreactivity?
[18082388] Curr Opin Immunol 20(1):105-10 (2008)

2010
1693
CSF-1, IGF-1, and the control of postnatal growth and development.
[20519640] J Leukoc Biol 88(3):475-81 (2010)

2010
1694
Molecular chaperones and protein-folding catalysts as intercellular signaling regulators in immunity and inflammation.
[20445014] J Leukoc Biol 88(3):445-62 (2010)

2010
1695
Endogenous ligands of TLR2 and TLR4: agonists or assistants?
[20179153] J Leukoc Biol 87(6):989-99 (2010)

2010
1696
The bone marrow: a site of neutrophil clearance.
[20483920] J Leukoc Biol 88(2):241-51 (2010)

2002
1697
Neutrophil-Kupffer cell interaction: a critical component of host defenses to systemic bacterial infections.
[12149414] J Leukoc Biol 72(2):239-48 (2002)

2010
1698
Editorial: PGE2-producing MDSC: a role in tumor progression?
[21041513] J Leukoc Biol 88(5):827-9 (2010)

2010
1699
Editorial: Are men rats? Dendritic cells in autoimmune glomerulonephritis.
[21041514] J Leukoc Biol 88(5):831-5 (2010)

2010
1700
Neutrophils and macrophages work in concert as inducers and effectors of adaptive immunity against extracellular and intracellular microbial pathogens.
[20110444] J Leukoc Biol 87(5):805-13 (2010)

2004
1701
Host defense function of the airway epithelium in health and disease: clinical background.
[12972516] J Leukoc Biol 75(1):5-17 (2004)

2004
1702
The chronic consequences of severe sepsis.
[14557384] J Leukoc Biol 75(3):408-12 (2004)

2010
1703
HVEM/LIGHT/BTLA/CD160 cosignaling pathways as targets for immune regulation.
[20007250] J Leukoc Biol 87(2):223-35 (2010)

2003
1704
Clearance of apoptotic cells: TGF-beta in the balance between inflammation and fibrosis.
[12960252] J Leukoc Biol 74(6):959-60 (2003)

2009
1705
Microglia: gatekeepers of central nervous system immunology.
[19028958] J Leukoc Biol 85(3):352-70 (2009)

2010
1706
CD57+ T lymphocytes and functional immune deficiency.
[19880576] J Leukoc Biol 87(1):107-16 (2010)

2010
1707
When two is better than one: macrophages and neutrophils work in concert in innate immunity as complementary and cooperative partners of a myeloid phagocyte system.
[20052802] J Leukoc Biol 87(1):93-106 (2010)

2010
1708
The battlefield of perforin/granzyme cell death pathways.
[19915166] J Leukoc Biol 87(2):237-43 (2010)

2009
1709
Review of the activation of TGF-beta in immunity.
[18818372] J Leukoc Biol 85(1):29-33 (2009)

2009
1710
Intact extracellular matrix and the maintenance of immune tolerance: high molecular weight hyaluronan promotes persistence of induced CD4+CD25+ regulatory T cells.
[19401397] J Leukoc Biol 86(3):567-72 (2009)

2009
1711
Interferon-lambdas: the modulators of antivirus, antitumor, and immune responses.
[19304895] J Leukoc Biol 86(1):23-32 (2009)

2009
1712
The endogenous Toll-like receptor 4 agonist S100A8/S100A9 (calprotectin) as innate amplifier of infection, autoimmunity, and cancer.
[19451397] J Leukoc Biol 86(3):557-66 (2009)

2009
1713
MAPK signaling pathways in the regulation of hematopoiesis.
[19498045] J Leukoc Biol 86(2):237-50 (2009)

2009
1714
Editorial: Hemopexin: newest member of the anti-inflammatory mediator club.
[19643739] J Leukoc Biol 86(2):203-4 (2009)

2009
1715
The role of circulating mesenchymal progenitor cells (fibrocytes) in the pathogenesis of pulmonary fibrosis.
[19581373] J Leukoc Biol 86(5):1111-8 (2009)

2004
1716
Biological applications of support vector machines.
[15606969] Brief Bioinform 5(4):328-38 (2004)

2008
1717
Facts from text: can text mining help to scale-up high-quality manual curation of gene products with ontologies?
[19060303] Brief Bioinform 9(6):466-78 (2008)

2010
1718
Advances in translational bioinformatics: computational approaches for the hunting of disease genes.
[20007728] Brief Bioinform 11(1):96-110 (2010)

2007
1719
Frontiers of biomedical text mining: current progress.
[17977867] Brief Bioinform 8(5):358-75 (2007)

2007
1720
A hitchhiker's guide to expressed sequence tag (EST) analysis.
[16772268] Brief Bioinform 8(1):6-21 (2007)

2007
1721
Partial least squares: a versatile tool for the analysis of high-dimensional genomic data.
[16772269] Brief Bioinform 8(1):32-44 (2007)

2009
1722
Expression profiling of microRNAs by deep sequencing.
[19332473] Brief Bioinform 10(5):490-7 (2009)

2007
1723
Methods and protocols for prediction of immunogenic epitopes.
[17077136] Brief Bioinform 8(2):96-108 (2007)

2007
1724
Evolving research trends in bioinformatics.
[17077138] Brief Bioinform 8(2):88-95 (2007)

2007
1725
Forensic DNA and bioinformatics.
[17384432] Brief Bioinform 8(2):117-28 (2007)

2007
1726
Bayeslan methods in bioinformatics and computational systems biology.
[17430978] Brief Bioinform 8(2):109-16 (2007)

2008
1727
Building a knowledge base for systems pathology.
[19073714] Brief Bioinform 9(6):518-31 (2008)

2005
1728
The many faces of sequence alignment.
[15826353] Brief Bioinform 6(1):6-22 (2005)

2005
1729
A Bayesian method for analysing spotted microarray data.
[16420731] Brief Bioinform 6(4):318-30 (2005)

2005
1730
Hairpins in bookstacks: information retrieval from biomedical text.
[16212771] Brief Bioinform 6(3):222-38 (2005)

2005   Text mining and ontologies in biomedicine: making sense of raw text.
1731   [16212772] Brief Bioinform 6(3):239-51 (2005)

2005   Information retrieval and knowledge discovery utilising a biomedical Semantic Web.
1732   [16212773] Brief Bioinform 6(3):252-62 (2005)

2005   Extraction of biological interaction networks from scientific literature.
1733   [16212774] Brief Bioinform 6(3):263-76 (2005)

2005   Online tools to support literature-based discovery in the life sciences.
1734   [16212775] Brief Bioinform 6(3):277-86 (2005)

2008   Protein structure databases with new web services for structural biology and biomedical research.
1735   [18430752] Brief Bioinform 9(4):276-85 (2008)

2008   Literature mining in support of drug discovery.
1736   [18820304] Brief Bioinform 9(6):479-92 (2008)

2010   The challenges of informatics in synthetic biology: from biomolecular networks to artificial organisms.
1737   [19906839] Brief Bioinform 11(1):80-95 (2010)

2008   Biomedical ontologies: a functional perspective.
1738   [18077472] Brief Bioinform 9(1):75-90 (2008)

2010   Cardiac output monitoring using indicator-dilution techniques: basics, limits, and perspectives.
1739   [20185659] Anesth Analg 110(3):799-811 (2010)

2007   Percussion pacing--an almost forgotten procedure for haemodynamically unstable bradycardias? A report of three case studies and review of the literature.
1740   [17327252] Br J Anaesth 98(4):429-33 (2007)

2006   Monitoring the injured brain: ICP and CBF.
1741   [16698860] Br J Anaesth 97(1):26-38 (2006)

2011   A review of current and emerging approaches to address failure-to-rescue.
1742   [21587063] Anesthesiology 115(2):421-31 (2011)

2011   Reducing noninfectious risks of blood transfusion.
1743   [21792054] Anesthesiology 115(3):635-49 (2011)

2011   Potential adverse ultrasound-related biological effects: a critical review.
1744   [21866043] Anesthesiology 115(5):1109-24 (2011)

2010   Pathophysiology and treatment of coagulopathy in massive hemorrhage and hemodilution.
1745   [20881594] Anesthesiology 113(5):1205-19 (2010)

2010   Role of transient receptor potential and acid-sensing ion channels in peripheral inflammatory pain.
1746   [20179512] Anesthesiology 112(3):729-41 (2010)

2011   Cardiopulmonary bypass-associated acute kidney injury.
1747   [21394005] Anesthesiology 114(4):964-70 (2011)

2004   Catecholamine-induced changes in the splanchnic circulation affecting systemic hemodynamics.
1748   [14739821] Anesthesiology 100(2):434-9 (2004)

2004   Mechanisms of cardioprotection by volatile anesthetics.
1749   [15108989] Anesthesiology 100(3):707-21 (2004)

2004
1750
Excitation-contraction coupling in the heart and the negative inotropic action of volatile anesthetics.
[15448535] Anesthesiology 101(4):999-1014 (2004)

2008
1751
Sympathetic nervous system: evaluation and importance for clinical general anesthesia.
[19034109] Anesthesiology 109(6):1113-31 (2008)

2007
1752
Diagnosis and treatment of vascular air embolism.
[17197859] Anesthesiology 106(1):164-77 (2007)

2009
1753
Massive blood transfusions: the impact of Vietnam military data on modern civilian transfusion medicine.
[19417598] Anesthesiology 110(6):1412-6 (2009)

2010
1754
Measles virus-induced suppression of immune responses.
[20636817] Immunol Rev 236(-):176-89 (2010)

2010
1755
Molecular mechanisms by which T-bet regulates T-helper cell commitment.
[20969596] Immunol Rev 238(1):233-46 (2010)

2010
1756
Lymphoid and myeloid lineage commitment in multipotent hematopoietic progenitors.
[20969583] Immunol Rev 238(1):37-46 (2010)

2010
1757
Mechanisms regulating dendritic cell specification and development.
[20969586] Immunol Rev 238(1):76-92 (2010)

2008
1758
Autoantibodies to tumor-associated antigens: reporters from the immune system.
[18364012] Immunol Rev 222(-):328-40 (2008)

2009
1759
RNA-based viral immunity initiated by the Dicer family of host immune receptors.
[19120484] Immunol Rev 227(1):176-88 (2009)

2009
1760
Autophagy and pattern recognition receptors in innate immunity.
[19120485] Immunol Rev 227(1):189-202 (2009)

2007
1761
PADB: published association database.
[17877839] BMC Bioinformatics 8(-):348 (2007)

2008
1762
GAPscreener: an automatic tool for screening human genetic association literature in PubMed using the support vector machine technique.
[18430222] BMC Bioinformatics 9(-):205 (2008)

2006
1763
The Autoimmune Disease Database: a dynamically compiled literature-derived database.
[16803617] BMC Bioinformatics 7(-):325 (2006)

2011
1764
The Global Evidence Mapping Initiative: scoping research in broad topic areas.
[21682870] BMC Med Res Methodol 11(-):92 (2011)

2009
1765
Lymphoid tissue inducer cells: architects of CD4 immune responses in mice and men.
[19659766] Clin Exp Immunol 157(1):20-6 (2009)

2010
1766
B7-h3 and its role in antitumor immunity.
[21127709] Clin Dev Immunol 2010(-):683875 (2010)

2010
1767
The initial immune reaction to a new tumor antigen is always stimulatory and probably necessary for the tumor's growth.
[20811480] Clin Dev Immunol 2010(-):- (2010)

2006
1768
Promiscuous gene expression in the thymus: the root of central tolerance.
[17162352] Clin Dev Immunol 13(2-4):81-99 (2006)

2010   **Signaling actions of electrophiles: anti-inflammatory therapeutic candidates.**
1769   [20124562] Mol Interv 10(1):39-50 (2010)

2005   **An extended vision for dynamic high-resolution intravital immune imaging.**
1770   [16216522] Semin Immunol 17(6):431-41 (2005)

2008   **Follicular dendritic cell networks of primary follicles and germinal centers: phenotype and function.**
1771   [18261920] Semin Immunol 20(1):14-25 (2008)

2008   **Ectopic lymphoid tissues and local immunity.**
1772   [18243731] Semin Immunol 20(1):26-42 (2008)

2008   **Germinal center structure and function: lessons from CD19.**
1773   [18243730] Semin Immunol 20(1):43-8 (2008)

2008   **The role of collagen deposition in depleting CD4+ T cells and limiting reconstitution in HIV-1 and**
1774   **SIV infections through damage to the secondary lymphoid organ niche.**
      [18595731] Semin Immunol 20(3):181-6 (2008)

2008   **T and B lymphocyte differentiation from hematopoietic stem cell.**
1775   [18583148] Semin Immunol 20(4):207-12 (2008)

2006   **Structural basis for recognition of MHC and MHC-like ligands by natural killer cell receptors.**
1776   [16737824] Semin Immunol 18(3):159-66 (2006)

2010   **Inflammatory mediators and insulin resistance in obesity: role of nuclear receptor signaling in**
1777   **macrophages.**
      [20508742] Mediators Inflamm 2010(-):219583 (2010)

2010   **Novel insights for systemic inflammation in sepsis and hemorrhage.**
1778   [20628562] Mediators Inflamm 2010(-):642462 (2010)

2010   **Modulation of Toll-like receptor activity by leukocyte Ig-like receptors and their effects during**
1779   **bacterial infection.**
      [20634939] Mediators Inflamm 2010(-):536478 (2010)

2010   **Macrophage migration inhibitory factor: critical role in obesity, insulin resistance, and associated**
1780   **comorbidities.**
      [20169173] Mediators Inflamm 2010(-):610479 (2010)

2010   **Matching therapy to body rhythms: an endocrine approach to treating rheumatoid arthritis.**
1781   [20889607] J Rheumatol 37(10):1981-2 (2010)

2011   **Enhancing single molecule imaging in optofluidics and microfluidics.**
1782   [21954349] Int J Mol Sci 12(8):5135-56 (2011)

2011   **Molecularly imprinted polymers: present and future prospective.**
1783   [22016636] Int J Mol Sci 12(9):5908-45 (2011)

2011   **Chaperoning roles of macromolecules interacting with proteins in vivo.**
1784   [21673934] Int J Mol Sci 12(3):1979-90 (2011)

2011   **Conformationally Constrained Histidines in the Design of Peptidomimetics: Strategies for the Ï‡-**
1785   **Space Control.**
      [21686155] Int J Mol Sci 12(5):2853-90 (2011)

2011   **Antioxidant properties of aminoethylcysteine ketimine decarboxylated dimer: a review.**
1786   [21686170] Int J Mol Sci 12(5):3072-84 (2011)

2011   **Multi-step usage of in vivo models during rational drug design and discovery.**
1787   [21731440] Int J Mol Sci 12(4):2262-74 (2011)

2011
1788
Functioning nanomachines seen in real-time in living bacteria using single-molecule and super-resolution fluorescence imaging.
[21731456] Int J Mol Sci 12(4):2518-42 (2011)

2010
1789
A review on progress in QSPR studies for surfactants.
[20479997] Int J Mol Sci 11(3):1020-47 (2010)

2010
1790
Matrix-assisted laser desorption/ionization imaging mass spectrometry.
[21614190] Int J Mol Sci 11(12):5040-55 (2010)

2010
1791
Quantum dots-from synthesis to applications in biomedicine and life sciences.
[20162007] Int J Mol Sci 11(1):154-63 (2010)

2009
1792
Quantum dots - characterization, preparation and usage in biological systems.
[19333427] Int J Mol Sci 10(2):656-73 (2009)

2008
1793
Selenium derivatization of nucleic acids for phase and structure determination in nucleic acid X-ray crystallography.
[19325748] Int J Mol Sci 9(3):258-71 (2008)

2011
1794
Congenitally corrected transposition.
[21569592] Orphanet J Rare Dis 6(-):22 (2011)

2011
1795
Therapy of Fabry disease with pharmacological chaperones: from in silico predictions to in vitro tests.
[22004918] Orphanet J Rare Dis 6(-):66 (2011)

2010
1796
Wolcott-Rallison syndrome.
[21050479] Orphanet J Rare Dis 5(-):29 (2010)

2010
1797
Expression of the disease on female carriers of X-linked lysosomal disorders: a brief review.
[20509947] Orphanet J Rare Dis 5(-):14 (2010)

2007
1798
Fibromuscular dysplasia.
[17555581] Orphanet J Rare Dis 2(-):28 (2007)

2011
1799
Ivermectin, 'wonder drug' from Japan: the human use perspective.
[21321478] Proc Jpn Acad Ser B Phys Biol Sci 87(2):13-28 (2011)

2010
1800
Development of fluorescent probes for bioimaging applications.
[20948177] Proc Jpn Acad Ser B Phys Biol Sci 86(8):837-47 (2010)

2010
1801
Conversion of brain cytosol profile from fetal to adult type during the perinatal period: taurine-NAA exchange.
[20551599] Proc Jpn Acad Ser B Phys Biol Sci 86(6):630-42 (2010)

2010
1802
Mechanisms of organelle division and inheritance and their implications regarding the origin of eukaryotic cells.
[20467212] Proc Jpn Acad Ser B Phys Biol Sci 86(5):455-71 (2010)

2010
1803
Phosphoinositide-binding interface proteins involved in shaping cell membranes.
[20467216] Proc Jpn Acad Ser B Phys Biol Sci 86(5):509-23 (2010)

2010
1804
Toward a superconducting quantum computer. Harnessing macroscopic quantum coherence.
[20431256] Proc Jpn Acad Ser B Phys Biol Sci 86(4):275-92 (2010)

2010
1805
Key structures of bacterial peptidoglycan and lipopolysaccharide triggering the innate immune system of higher animals: chemical synthesis and functional studies.
[20431259] Proc Jpn Acad Ser B Phys Biol Sci 86(4):322-37 (2010)

2010
1806
Molecular approach to human leukemia: isolation and characterization of the first human retrovirus HTLV-1 and its impact on tumorigenesis in adult T-cell leukemia.
[20154469] Proc Jpn Acad Ser B Phys Biol Sci 86(2):117-30 (2010)

2010
1807
Laser acceleration and its future.
[20228616] Proc Jpn Acad Ser B Phys Biol Sci 86(3):147-57 (2010)

2010
1808
Spectroscopy of antiprotonic helium atoms and its contribution to the fundamental physical constants.
[20075605] Proc Jpn Acad Ser B Phys Biol Sci 86(1):1-10 (2010)

2009
1809
The proteasome: overview of structure and functions.
[19145068] Proc Jpn Acad Ser B Phys Biol Sci 85(1):12-36 (2009)

2009
1810
Raman tensors and their application in structural studies of biological systems.
[19282645] Proc Jpn Acad Ser B Phys Biol Sci 85(3):83-97 (2009)

2008
1811
Glycine cleavage system: reaction mechanism, physiological significance, and hyperglycinemia.
[18941301] Proc Jpn Acad Ser B Phys Biol Sci 84(7):246-63 (2008)

2008
1812
Platelet aggregation in the formation of tumor metastasis.
[18941298] Proc Jpn Acad Ser B Phys Biol Sci 84(6):189-98 (2008)

2008
1813
From designer Lewis acid to designer BrÃ‚nsted acid towards more reactive and selective acid catalysis.
[18941293] Proc Jpn Acad Ser B Phys Biol Sci 84(5):134-46 (2008)

2008
1814
Total synthesis and development of bioactive natural products.
[18941289] Proc Jpn Acad Ser B Phys Biol Sci 84(4):87-106 (2008)

2008
1815
Evolving genetic code.
[18941287] Proc Jpn Acad Ser B Phys Biol Sci 84(2):58-74 (2008)

2010
1816
A window into third-generation sequencing.
[20858600] Hum Mol Genet 19(R2):R227-40 (2010)

2011
1817
Cellular toxicity of expanded RNA repeats: focus on RNA foci.
[21729883] Hum Mol Genet 20(19):3811-21 (2011)

2010
1818
Allele-specific and heritable chromatin signatures in humans.
[20846943] Hum Mol Genet 19(R2):R204-9 (2010)

2010
1819
Allele-specific DNA methylation: beyond imprinting.
[20855472] Hum Mol Genet 19(R2):R210-20 (2010)

2010
1820
Small insertions and deletions (INDELs) in human genomes.
[20858594] Hum Mol Genet 19(R2):R131-6 (2010)

2010
1821
Fine-scale population structure and the era of next-generation sequencing.
[20876616] Hum Mol Genet 19(R2):R221-6 (2010)

2010
1822
Evolutionary history of regulatory variation in human populations.
[20876617] Hum Mol Genet 19(R2):R197-203 (2010)

2010
1823
Exome sequencing: the sweet spot before whole genomes.
[20705737] Hum Mol Genet 19(R2):R145-51 (2010)

2010
1824
Large non-coding RNAs: missing links in cancer?
[20729297] Hum Mol Genet 19(R2):R152-61 (2010)

2010   Transcribed dark matter: meaning or myth?
1825   [20798109] Hum Mol Genet 19(R2):R162-8 (2010)

2010   Synthetic associations in the context of genome-wide association scan signals.
1826   [20805105] Hum Mol Genet 19(R2):R137-44 (2010)

2010   Loss-of-function variants in the genomes of healthy humans.
1827   [20805107] Hum Mol Genet 19(R2):R125-30 (2010)

2010   Phenotypic variability and genetic susceptibility to genomic disorders.
1828   [20807775] Hum Mol Genet 19(R2):R176-87 (2010)

2010   Analysis of next-generation genomic data in cancer: accomplishments and challenges.
1829   [20843826] Hum Mol Genet 19(R2):R188-96 (2010)

2010   Massively parallel sequencing and rare disease.
1830   [20846941] Hum Mol Genet 19(R2):R119-24 (2010)

2010   Partners in crime: bidirectional transcription in unstable microsatellite disease.
1831   [20368264] Hum Mol Genet 19(R1):R77-82 (2010)

2010
1832   A pivotal role for PINK1 and autophagy in mitochondrial quality control: implications for Parkinson disease.
   [20385539] Hum Mol Genet 19(R1):R28-37 (2010)

2007   Copy-number variation in control population cohorts.
1833   [17911159] Hum Mol Genet 16 Spec No. 2(-):R168-73 (2007)

2007   The origin of human aneuploidy: where we have been, where we are going.
1834   [17911163] Hum Mol Genet 16 Spec No. 2(-):R203-8 (2007)

2007   Epigenetic gene silencing in cancer: the DNA hypermethylome.
1835   [17613547] Hum Mol Genet 16 Spec No 1(-):R50-9 (2007)

2009
1836   Evaluation of imputation-based association in and around the integrin-alpha-M (ITGAM) gene and replication of robust association between a non-synonymous functional variant within ITGAM and systemic lupus erythematosus (SLE).
   [19129174] Hum Mol Genet 18(6):1171-80 (2009)

2009   Lessons learnt from large-scale exon re-sequencing of the X chromosome.
1837   [19297402] Hum Mol Genet 18(R1):R60-4 (2009)

2009   Constitutional aneuploidy and cancer predisposition.
1838   [19297405] Hum Mol Genet 18(R1):R84-93 (2009)

2009   Copy number variants, diseases and gene expression.
1839   [19297395] Hum Mol Genet 18(R1):R1-8 (2009)

2008   Skin and hair: models for exploring organ regeneration.
1840   [18632698] Hum Mol Genet 17(R1):R54-9 (2008)

2008   Extending genome-wide association studies to copy-number variation.
1841   [18852202] Hum Mol Genet 17(R2):R135-42 (2008)

2008   Using gene expression to investigate the genetic basis of complex disorders.
1842   [18852201] Hum Mol Genet 17(R2):R129-34 (2008)

2008   Practical aspects of imputation-driven meta-analysis of genome-wide association studies.
1843   [18852200] Hum Mol Genet 17(R2):R122-8 (2008)

2009   **The resolution of the genetics of gene expression.**
1844   [19808798] Hum Mol Genet 18(R2):R211-5 (2009)

2009   **Cancer genome sequencing: a review.**
1845   [19808792] Hum Mol Genet 18(R2):R163-8 (2009)

2009   **Aicardi-Goutieres syndrome and related phenotypes: linking nucleic acid metabolism with**
1846   **autoimmunity.**
     [19808788] Hum Mol Genet 18(R2):R130-6 (2009)

2006   **An introduction to the Semantic Web for health sciences librarians.**
1847   [16636713] J Med Libr Assoc 94(2):198-205 (2006)

2011   **The impact of free access to the scientific literature: a review of recent research.**
1848   [21753913] J Med Libr Assoc 99(3):208-17 (2011)

2006   **Open access: implications for scholarly publishing and medical libraries.**
1849   [16888657] J Med Libr Assoc 94(3):253-62 (2006)

2007   **Epigenetics in male germ cells.**
1850   [17287457] J Androl 28(4):466-80 (2007)

2010   **Re-valuing the amygdala.**
1851   [20299204] Curr Opin Neurobiol 20(2):221-30 (2010)

2010   **Prefrontal control of fear: more than just extinction.**
1852   [20303254] Curr Opin Neurobiol 20(2):231-5 (2010)

2010   **Synchronous neural activity and memory formation.**
1853   [20303255] Curr Opin Neurobiol 20(2):150-5 (2010)

2004   **Fiber optic in vivo imaging in the mammalian nervous system.**
1854   [15464896] Curr Opin Neurobiol 14(5):617-28 (2004)

2007   **From chills to chilis: mechanisms for thermosensation and chemesthesis via thermoTRPs.**
1855   [17706410] Curr Opin Neurobiol 17(4):490-7 (2007)

2007   **Visualizing circuits and systems using transgenic reporters of neural activity.**
1856   [18036810] Curr Opin Neurobiol 17(5):567-71 (2007)

2007   **Circuit reconstruction tools today.**
1857   [18082394] Curr Opin Neurobiol 17(5):601-8 (2007)

2009   **Caenorhabditis elegans pheromones regulate multiple complex behaviors.**
1858   [19665885] Curr Opin Neurobiol 19(4):378-88 (2009)

2008   **Fear, faces, and the human amygdala.**
1859   [18655833] Curr Opin Neurobiol 18(2):166-72 (2008)

2008   **Nerve injury signaling.**
1860   [18655834] Curr Opin Neurobiol 18(3):276-83 (2008)

2002   **DNA methylation patterns and epigenetic memory.**
1861   [11782440] Genes Dev 16(1):6-21 (2002)

2011   **CpG islands and the regulation of transcription.**
1862   [21576262] Genes Dev 25(10):1010-22 (2011)

2011   **Ending the message: poly(A) signals then and now.**
1863   [21896654] Genes Dev 25(17):1770-82 (2011)

2010   **Cytidine deaminases: AIDing DNA demethylation?**
1864   [20889711] Genes Dev 24(19):2107-14 (2010)

2010   **Induced pluripotency: history, mechanisms, and applications.**
1865   [20952534] Genes Dev 24(20):2239-63 (2010)

2010   **Eph/ephrin molecules--a hub for signaling and endocytosis.**
1866   [21078817] Genes Dev 24(22):2480-92 (2010)

2010   **How does the royal family of Tudor rule the PIWI-interacting RNA pathway?**
1867   [20360382] Genes Dev 24(7):636-46 (2010)

2010   **GEN1/Yen1 and the SLX4 complex: Solutions to the problem of Holliday junction resolution.**
1868   [20203129] Genes Dev 24(6):521-36 (2010)

2010   **Coordinating cohesion, co-orientation, and congression during meiosis: lessons from holocentric chromosomes.**
1869   [20123904] Genes Dev 24(3):219-28 (2010)

2007   **The origins of oncomice: a history of the first transgenic mice genetically engineered to develop cancer.**
1870   [17875663] Genes Dev 21(18):2258-70 (2007)

2008   **Riboswitch RNAs: using RNA to sense cellular metabolism.**
1871   [19141470] Genes Dev 22(24):3383-90 (2008)

2009   **Tumor suppressors and cell metabolism: a recipe for cancer growth.**
1872   [19270154] Genes Dev 23(5):537-48 (2009)

2009   **Positioning cytokinesis.**
1873   [19299557] Genes Dev 23(6):660-74 (2009)

2009   **An operational definition of epigenetics.**
1874   [19339683] Genes Dev 23(7):781-3 (2009)

2009   **Current-generation high-throughput sequencing: deepening insights into mammalian transcriptomes.**
1875   [19528315] Genes Dev 23(12):1379-86 (2009)

2009   **The pathophysiology of mitochondrial disease as modeled in the mouse.**
1876   [19651984] Genes Dev 23(15):1714-36 (2009)

2005   **Poly(ADP-ribosyl)ation by PARP-1: 'PAR-laying' NAD+ into a nuclear signal.**
1877   [16140981] Genes Dev 19(17):1951-67 (2005)

2008   **Migratory neighbors and distant invaders: tumor-associated niche cells.**
1878   [18316475] Genes Dev 22(5):559-74 (2008)

2008   **Signal integration in bacterial two-component regulatory systems.**
1879   [18832064] Genes Dev 22(19):2601-11 (2008)

2005   **Dynamic molecular linkers of the genome: the first decade of SMC proteins.**
1880   [15937217] Genes Dev 19(11):1269-87 (2005)

2009   **Evolutionary conservation and adaptation in the mechanism that regulates SREBP action: what a long, strange tRIP it's been.**
1881   [19933148] Genes Dev 23(22):2578-91 (2009)

2009   **Endoreplication: polyploidy with purpose.**
1882   [19884253] Genes Dev 23(21):2461-77 (2009)

2009 **Genomic imprinting: employing and avoiding epigenetic processes.**
1883   [19759261] Genes Dev 23(18):2124-33 (2009)

2009 **Long noncoding RNAs: functional surprises from the RNA world.**
1884   [19571179] Genes Dev 23(13):1494-504 (2009)

2006 **Dosage compensation in mammals: fine-tuning the expression of the X chromosome.**
1885   [16847345] Genes Dev 20(14):1848-67 (2006)

2010 **Optimizing copy number variation analysis using genome-wide short sequence oligonucleotide arrays.**
1886   [20156996] Nucleic Acids Res 38(10):3275-86 (2010)

2002 **Evaluation of sequence motifs found in scaffold/matrix-attached regions (S/MARs).**
1887   [12140328] Nucleic Acids Res 30(15):3433-42 (2002)

2002 **Having it both ways: transcription factors that bind DNA and RNA.**
1888   [12364590] Nucleic Acids Res 30(19):4118-26 (2002)

2011 **How does DNA break during chromosomal translocations?**
1889   [21498543] Nucleic Acids Res 39(14):5813-25 (2011)

2011 **Bovine Genome Database: integrated tools for genome annotation and discovery.**
1890   [21123190] Nucleic Acids Res 39(Database issue):D830-4 (2011)

2011 **Efficient design and assembly of custom TALEN and other TAL effector-based constructs for DNA targeting.**
1891   [21493687] Nucleic Acids Res 39(12):e82 (2011)

2011 **DNA translocation by type III restriction enzymes: a comparison of current models of their operation derived from ensemble and single-molecule measurements.**
1892   [21310716] Nucleic Acids Res 39(11):4525-31 (2011)

2011 **Handpicking epigenetic marks with PHD fingers.**
1893   [21813457] Nucleic Acids Res 39(21):9061-71 (2011)

2011 **Transcription factories in the context of the nuclear and genome organization.**
1894   [21880598] Nucleic Acids Res 39(21):9085-92 (2011)

2011 **Quantification noise in single cell experiments.**
1895   [21745823] Nucleic Acids Res 39(18):e124 (2011)

2011 **Genome-wide analysis of the relationships between DNaseI HS, histone modifications and gene expression reveals distinct modes of chromatin domains.**
1896   [21685456] Nucleic Acids Res 39(17):7428-43 (2011)

2011 **Functional regulation of FEN1 nuclease and its link to cancer.**
1897   [20929870] Nucleic Acids Res 39(3):781-94 (2011)

2011 **Towards BioDBcore: a community-defined information specification for biological databases.**
1898   [21097465] Nucleic Acids Res 39(Database issue):D7-10 (2011)

2011 **NCBI GEO: archive for functional genomics data sets--10 years on.**
1899   [21097893] Nucleic Acids Res 39(Database issue):D1005-10 (2011)

2011 **OMA 2011: orthology inference among 1000 complete genomes.**
1900   [21113020] Nucleic Acids Res 39(Database issue):D289-94 (2011)

2010 **InTERTpreting telomerase structure and function.**
1901   [20460453] Nucleic Acids Res 38(17):5609-22 (2010)

2004   **Comprehensive comparison of six microarray technologies.**
1902   [15333675] Nucleic Acids Res 32(15):e124 (2004)

2010   **DNA supercoiling and its role in DNA decatenation and unknotting.**
1903   [20026582] Nucleic Acids Res 38(7):2119-33 (2010)

2010   **Molecular mechanisms of eukaryotic pre-mRNA 3' end processing regulation.**
1904   [20044349] Nucleic Acids Res 38(9):2757-74 (2010)

2003   **Unusual DNA duplex and hairpin motifs.**
1905   [12736295] Nucleic Acids Res 31(10):2461-74 (2003)

2007   **eTBLAST: a web server to identify expert reviewers, appropriate journals and similar publications.**
1906   [17452348] Nucleic Acids Res 35(Web Server issue):W12-5 (2007)

2008   **See me, feel me: methods to concurrently visualize and manipulate single DNA molecules and**
1907   **associated proteins.**
        [18586820] Nucleic Acids Res 36(13):4381-9 (2008)

2010   **Sequence-non-specific effects of RNA interference triggers and microRNA regulators.**
1908   [19843612] Nucleic Acids Res 38(1):1-16 (2010)

2010   **All things must pass: contrasts and commonalities in eukaryotic and bacterial mRNA decay.**
1909   [20520623] Nat Rev Mol Cell Biol 11(7):467-78 (2010)

2010   **The prion hypothesis: from biological anomaly to basic regulatory mechanism.**
1910   [21081963] Nat Rev Mol Cell Biol 11(12):823-33 (2010)

2010   **A nucleator arms race: cellular control of actin assembly.**
1911   [20237478] Nat Rev Mol Cell Biol 11(4):237-51 (2010)

2008   **Shaping cups into phagosomes and macropinosomes.**
1912   [18612320] Nat Rev Mol Cell Biol 9(8):639-49 (2008)

2010   **Genome destabilization by homologous recombination in the germ line.**
1913   [20164840] Nat Rev Mol Cell Biol 11(3):182-95 (2010)

2009   **The 3Ms of central spindle assembly: microtubules, motors and MAPs.**
1914   [19197328] Nat Rev Mol Cell Biol 10(1):9-20 (2009)

2009   **Ion channels versus ion pumps: the principal difference, in principle.**
1915   [19339978] Nat Rev Mol Cell Biol 10(5):344-52 (2009)

2009   **Ubiquitin-like protein activation by E1 enzymes: the apex for downstream signalling pathways.**
1916   [19352404] Nat Rev Mol Cell Biol 10(5):319-31 (2009)

2008   **The Rpd3/Hda1 family of lysine deacetylases: from bacteria and yeast to mice and men.**
1917   [18292778] Nat Rev Mol Cell Biol 9(3):206-18 (2008)

2008   **How to succeed in science: a concise guide for young biomedical scientists. Part II: making**
1918   **discoveries.**
        [18401347] Nat Rev Mol Cell Biol 9(6):491-4 (2008)

2008   **Phagosome maturation: going through the acid test.**
1919   [18813294] Nat Rev Mol Cell Biol 9(10):781-95 (2008)

2008   **Design principles of biochemical oscillators.**
1920   [18971947] Nat Rev Mol Cell Biol 9(12):981-91 (2008)

2009   **Endocytosis and signalling: intertwining molecular networks.**
1921   [19696798] Nat Rev Mol Cell Biol 10(9):609-22 (2009)

2003   **Molecular mechanisms of irradiation-induced apoptosis.**
1922   [12456331] Front Biosci 8(-):d9-19 (2003)

2009   **Depression and pain.**
1923   [19482603] Front Biosci 14(-):5031-51 (2009)

2009   **Neurobiology of depression, fibromyalgia and neuropathic pain.**
1924   [19482616] Front Biosci 14(-):5291-338 (2009)

2008   **Prolyl 4-hydroxylase activity-responsive transcription factors: from hydroxylation to gene**
1925   **expression and neuroprotection.**
        [17981760] Front Biosci 13(-):2875-87 (2008)

2008   **The role of purinergic signaling in the liver and in transplantation: effects of extracellular**
1926   **nucleotides on hepatic graft vascular injury, rejection and metabolism.**
        [17981736] Front Biosci 13(-):2588-603 (2008)

2009   **Targeting the AMPK pathway for the treatment of Type 2 diabetes.**
1927   [19273282] Front Biosci 14(-):3380-400 (2009)

2009   **The inflammatory network: bridging senescent stroma and epithelial tumorigenesis.**
1928   [19273333] Front Biosci 14(-):4044-57 (2009)

2009   **The collagen receptor uPARAP/Endo180.**
1929   [19273187] Front Biosci 14(-):2103-14 (2009)

2010   **D-chiro-inositol glycans in insulin signaling and insulin resistance.**
1930   [20811656] Mol Med 16(11-12):543-52 (2010)

2011   **New insights of an old defense system: structure, function, and clinical relevance of the complement**
1931   **system.**
        [21046060] Mol Med 17(3-4):317-29 (2011)

2011   **A paradoxical role for myeloid-derived suppressor cells in sepsis and trauma.**
1932   [21085745] Mol Med 17(3-4):281-92 (2011)

2010   **A new view of carcinogenesis and an alternative approach to cancer therapy.**
1933   [20062820] Mol Med 16(3-4):144-53 (2010)

2003   **The cholinergic anti-inflammatory pathway: a missing link in neuroimmunomodulation.**
1934   [14571320] Mol Med 9(5-8):125-34 (2003)

2009   **Melatonin: an established antioxidant worthy of use in clinical trials.**
1935   [19011689] Mol Med 15(1-2):43-50 (2009)

2010   **RNA surveillance: molecular approaches in transcript quality control and their implications in clinical**
1936   **diseases.**
        [19829759] Mol Med 16(1-2):53-68 (2010)

2010   **Ghrelin as a novel therapy for radiation combined injury.**
1937   [20101281] Mol Med 16(3-4):137-43 (2010)

2010   **The ANG-(1-7)/ACE2/mas axis in the regulation of nephron function.**
1938   [20375118] Am J Physiol Renal Physiol 298(6):F1297-305 (2010)

2010   **Regulated oxygen sensing by protein hydroxylation in renal erythropoietin-producing cells.**
1939   [20219824] Am J Physiol Renal Physiol 298(6):F1287-96 (2010)

2002 **Extracellular cAMP inhibits proximal reabsorption: are plasma membrane cAMP receptors involved?**
1940 [11832418] Am J Physiol Renal Physiol 282(3):F376-92 (2002)

2002 **Xenotransplantation of developing kidneys.**
1941 [12217850] Am J Physiol Renal Physiol 283(4):F601-6 (2002)

2004 **Hepatocyte growth factor in kidney fibrosis: therapeutic potential and mechanisms of action.**
1942 [15180923] Am J Physiol Renal Physiol 287(1):F7-16 (2004)

2003 **Natriuretic peptides and acute renal failure.**
1943 [12842858] Am J Physiol Renal Physiol 285(2):F167-77 (2003)

2007 **Assessment of renal autoregulation.**
1944 [17229679] Am J Physiol Renal Physiol 292(4):F1105-23 (2007)

2007 **Uncoupling of the VEGF-endothelial nitric oxide axis in diabetic nephropathy: an explanation for the**
1945 **paradoxical effects of VEGF in renal disease.**
  [17545302] Am J Physiol Renal Physiol 292(6):F1665-72 (2007)

2009 **Vascular consequences of dietary salt intake.**
1946 [19339634] Am J Physiol Renal Physiol 297(2):F237-43 (2009)

2009 **Gap junctional intercellular communication in the juxtaglomerular apparatus.**
1947 [19073638] Am J Physiol Renal Physiol 296(5):F939-46 (2009)

2009 **A comprehensive guide to the ROMK potassium channel: form and function in health and disease.**
1948 [19458126] Am J Physiol Renal Physiol 297(4):F849-63 (2009)

2009 **The thiazide-sensitive Na+-Cl- cotransporter: molecular biology, functional properties, and**
1949 **regulation by WNKs.**
  [19474192] Am J Physiol Renal Physiol 297(4):F838-48 (2009)

2009 **Regulation of mRNA translation in renal physiology and disease.**
1950 [19535566] Am J Physiol Renal Physiol 297(5):F1153-65 (2009)

2010 **Physiology and pathophysiology of the calcium-sensing receptor in the kidney.**
1951 [19923405] Am J Physiol Renal Physiol 298(3):F485-99 (2010)

2009 **Heme oxygenase: the key to renal function regulation.**
1952 [19570878] Am J Physiol Renal Physiol 297(5):F1137-52 (2009)

2009 **Cell biology and physiology of the uroepithelium.**
1953 [19587142] Am J Physiol Renal Physiol 297(6):F1477-501 (2009)

2009 **Renal tubulointerstitial fibrosis: common but never simple.**
1954 [19144691] Am J Physiol Renal Physiol 296(6):F1239-44 (2009)

2009 **TRPMLs: in sickness and in health.**
1955 [19158345] Am J Physiol Renal Physiol 296(6):F1245-54 (2009)

2010 **Reciprocal control of 1,25-dihydroxyvitamin D and FGF23 formation involving the FGF23/Klotho**
1956 **system.**
  [20798257] Clin J Am Soc Nephrol 5(9):1717-22 (2010)

2010 **Fibroblast growth factor 23 and disordered vitamin D metabolism in chronic kidney disease:**
1957 **updating the "trade-off" hypothesis.**
  [20507957] Clin J Am Soc Nephrol 5(9):1710-6 (2010)

2010 **Topics in transplantation medicine for general nephrologists.**
1958 [20576830] Clin J Am Soc Nephrol 5(8):1518-29 (2010)

2010
1959
Circulating permeability factors in idiopathic nephrotic syndrome and focal segmental glomerulosclerosis.
[20966123] Clin J Am Soc Nephrol 5(11):2115-21 (2010)

2010
1960
Risk factors associated with patency loss of hemodialysis vascular access within 6 months.
[20576823] Clin J Am Soc Nephrol 5(10):1787-92 (2010)

2010
1961
Potassium homeostasis and renin-angiotensin-aldosterone system inhibitors.
[20150448] Clin J Am Soc Nephrol 5(3):531-48 (2010)

2010
1962
Familial renal glucosuria and SGLT2: from a mendelian trait to a therapeutic target.
[19965550] Clin J Am Soc Nephrol 5(1):133-41 (2010)

2010
1963
Paraneoplastic syndromes and the kidney.
[20228504] Saudi J Kidney Dis Transpl 21(2):222-31 (2010)

2010
1964
Renal thrombotic microangiopathy revisited: when a lesion is not a clinical finding.
[20427860] Saudi J Kidney Dis Transpl 21(3):411-6 (2010)

2004
1965
Activation and modulation of ligand-gated ion channels.
[15119941] Physiol Res 53 Suppl 1(-):S103-13 (2004)

2010
1966
Analysis of the electrical heart field.
[20626216] Physiol Res 59 Suppl 1(-):S19-24 (2010)

2010
1967
Measurement of cellular excitability by whole cell patch clamp technique.
[20626213] Physiol Res 59 Suppl 1(-):S1-7 (2010)

2010
1968
New insights into application of cardiac monophasic action potential.
[20406044] Physiol Res 59(5):645-50 (2010)

2010
1969
Application of proteomics in biomarker discovery: a primer for the clinician.
[19929137] Physiol Res 59(4):471-97 (2010)

2010
1970
Glycotoxines, carbonyl stress and relevance to diabetes and its complications.
[19537931] Physiol Res 59(2):147-56 (2010)

2010
1971
New insights into mechanisms of atrial fibrillation.
[19249911] Physiol Res 59(1):1-12 (2010)

2010
1972
The role of renin-angiotensin system in prothrombotic state in essential hypertension.
[19249905] Physiol Res 59(1):13-23 (2010)

2007
1973
Biochemical and biophysical aspects of collagen nanostructure in the extracellular matrix.
[17552894] Physiol Res 56 Suppl 1(-):S51-60 (2007)

2009
1974
End-organ damage in hypertensive transgenic Ren-2 rats: influence of early and late endothelin receptor blockade.
[20131938] Physiol Res 58 Suppl 2(-):S69-78 (2009)

2009
1975
Fibroblast growth factor 21: a novel metabolic regulator with potential therapeutic properties in obesity/type 2 diabetes mellitus.
[19331512] Physiol Res 58(1):1-7 (2009)

2008
1976
14-3-3 proteins: a family of versatile molecular regulators.
[18481918] Physiol Res 57 Suppl 3(-):S11-21 (2008)

2008
1977
Calcium-dependent desensitization of vanilloid receptor TRPV1: a mechanism possibly involved in analgesia induced by topical application of capsaicin.
[18481914] Physiol Res 57 Suppl 3(-):S59-68 (2008)

2008   **Pathological potential of astroglia.**
1978   [18481910] Physiol Res 57 Suppl 3(-):S101-10 (2008)

2008   **Mechanisms of neurogenic pulmonary edema development.**
1979   [18052674] Physiol Res 57(4):499-506 (2008)

2008   **Neurobiological aspects of depressive disorder and antidepressant treatment: role of glia.**
1980   [17465696] Physiol Res 57(2):151-64 (2008)

2008   **Postoperative delirium in the elderly: diagnosis and management.**
1981   [18686756] Clin Interv Aging 3(2):351-5 (2008)

2011   **Sepsis-associated encephalopathy: not just delirium.**
1982   [22012058] Clinics (Sao Paulo) 66(10):1825-31 (2011)

2008   **Sepsis: from bench to bedside.**
1983   [18297215] Clinics (Sao Paulo) 63(1):109-20 (2008)

2011   **Genome diagnostics: next-generation sequencing, new genome-wide association studies and clinical challenges.**
1984   [21902524] Expert Rev Mol Diagn 11(7):663-6 (2011)

2010   **Great expectations: using massively parallel sequencing to solve inherited disorders.**
1985   [20964599] Expert Rev Mol Diagn 10(7):833-6 (2010)

2010   **Bone marrow microenvironment in myelomagenesis: its potential role in early diagnosis.**
1986   [20465501] Expert Rev Mol Diagn 10(4):465-80 (2010)

2010   **DNA methylation as a universal biomarker.**
1987   [20465502] Expert Rev Mol Diagn 10(4):481-8 (2010)

2007   **Drug discovery without a molecular target: the road less traveled.**
1988   [17187477] Expert Rev Mol Diagn 7(1):1-4 (2007)

2009   **Nonsense-mediated decay: linking a basic cellular process to human disease.**
1989   [19435450] Expert Rev Mol Diagn 9(4):299-303 (2009)

2009   **Molecular copy-number counting: potential of single-molecule diagnostics.**
1990   [19435452] Expert Rev Mol Diagn 9(4):309-12 (2009)

2003   **Cellular zinc and redox states converge in the metallothionein/thionein pair.**
1991   [12730443] J Nutr 133(5 Suppl 1):1460S-2S (2003)

2010   **The developmental origins, mechanisms, and implications of metabolic syndrome.**
1992   [20107145] J Nutr 140(3):648-52 (2010)

2007   **Aromatic L-amino acids activate the calcium-sensing receptor.**
1993   [17513419] J Nutr 137(6 Suppl 1):1524S-1527S; discussion 1548S (2007)

2007   **Tyrosine, phenylalanine, and catecholamine synthesis and function in the brain.**
1994   [17513421] J Nutr 137(6 Suppl 1):1539S-1547S; discussion 1548S (2007)

2009   **Repression of transposable elements by histone biotinylation.**
1995   [19812216] J Nutr 139(12):2389-92 (2009)

2006   **The many facets of hyperhomocysteinemia: studies from the Framingham cohorts.**
1996   [16702347] J Nutr 136(6 Suppl):1726S-1730S (2006)

2006   **Mammalian cysteine metabolism: new insights into regulation of cysteine metabolism.**
1997   [16702335] J Nutr 136(6 Suppl):1652S-1659S (2006)

2006 **The sulfur-containing amino acids: an overview.**
1998   [16702333] J Nutr 136(6 Suppl):1636S-1640S (2006)

2010 **Live cell imaging of mechanotransduction.**
1999   [20356874] J R Soc Interface 7 Suppl 3(-):S365-75 (2010)

2010 **Mechanosensitivity of ion channels based on protein-lipid interactions.**
2000   [20356872] J R Soc Interface 7 Suppl 3(-):S307-20 (2010)

2010 **Single cell optical transfection.**
2001   [20064901] J R Soc Interface 7(47):863-71 (2010)

2010 **Surface-enhanced Raman scattering biomedical applications of plasmonic colloidal particles.**
2002   [20462878] J R Soc Interface 7 Suppl 4(-):S435-50 (2010)

2010 **Fluorescence-based transient state monitoring for biomolecular spectroscopy and imaging.**
2003   [20375039] J R Soc Interface 7(49):1135-44 (2010)

2011 **Scanning ion conductance microscopy: a convergent high-resolution technology for multi-**
2004   **parametric analysis of living cardiovascular cells.**
        [21325316] J R Soc Interface 8(60):913-25 (2011)

2010 **Electrophoretic deposition of biomaterials.**
2005   [20504802] J R Soc Interface 7 Suppl 5(-):S581-613 (2010)

2005 **Statistical geometry of pores and statistics of porous nanofibrous assemblies.**
2006   [16849188] J R Soc Interface 2(4):309-18 (2005)

2008 **Biological switches and clocks.**
2007   [18522926] J R Soc Interface 5 Suppl 1(-):S1-8 (2008)

2008 **Development of free-energy-based models for chaperonin containing TCP-1 mediated folding of**
2008   **actin.**
        [18708324] J R Soc Interface 5(29):1391-408 (2008)

2010 **Avian magnetite-based magnetoreception: a physiologist's perspective.**
2009   [20106875] J R Soc Interface 7 Suppl 2(-):S193-205 (2010)

2010 **Magnetoreception in eusocial insects: an update.**
2010   [20106876] J R Soc Interface 7 Suppl 2(-):S207-25 (2010)

2010 **Photoreceptor-based magnetoreception: optimal design of receptor molecules, cells, and neuronal**
2011   **processing.**
        [20129953] J R Soc Interface 7 Suppl 2(-):S135-46 (2010)

2010 **Optical imaging-guided cancer therapy with fluorescent nanoparticles.**
2012   [19759055] J R Soc Interface 7(42):3-18 (2010)

2007 **Biology by design: reduction and synthesis of cellular components and behaviour.**
2013   [17251159] J R Soc Interface 4(15):607-23 (2007)

2009 **Harnessing nature's toolbox: regulatory elements for synthetic biology.**
2014   [19324675] J R Soc Interface 6 Suppl 4(-):S535-46 (2009)

2009 **You're one in a googol: optimizing genes for protein expression.**
2015   [19324676] J R Soc Interface 6 Suppl 4(-):S467-76 (2009)

2009 **Challenges in the computational design of proteins.**
2016   [19324680] J R Soc Interface 6 Suppl 4(-):S477-91 (2009)

2009   **Bioinspired interface for nanobiodevices based on phospholipid polymer chemistry.**
2017   [19324688] J R Soc Interface 6 Suppl 3(-):S279-91 (2009)

2009   **Intelligently deciphering unintelligible designs: algorithmic algebraic model checking in systems biology.**
2018   [19364723] J R Soc Interface 6(36):575-97 (2009)

2009   **Rastering strategy for screening and centring of microcrystal samples of human membrane proteins with a sub-10 microm size X-ray synchrotron beam.**
2019   [19535414] J R Soc Interface 6 Suppl 5(-):S587-97 (2009)

2009   **Neutrons for biologists: a beginner's guide, or why you should consider using neutrons.**
2020   [19656821] J R Soc Interface 6 Suppl 5(-):S567-73 (2009)

2009   **Interfacial assembly of proteins and peptides: recent examples studied by neutron reflection.**
2021   [19656822] J R Soc Interface 6 Suppl 5(-):S659-70 (2009)

2008   **Automatic identification of bird targets with radar via patterns produced by wing flapping.**
2022   [18331979] J R Soc Interface 5(26):1041-53 (2008)

2008   **Current techniques for single-cell lysis.**
2023   [18426769] J R Soc Interface 5 Suppl 2(-):S131-8 (2008)

2010   **Lipid bilayer regulation of membrane protein function: gramicidin channels as molecular force probes.**
2024   [19940001] J R Soc Interface 7(44):373-95 (2010)

2010   **Cryptochromes--a potential magnetoreceptor: what do we know and what do we want to know?**
2025   [19906675] J R Soc Interface 7 Suppl 2(-):S147-62 (2010)

2009   **Atomic-scale dynamics inside living cells explored by neutron scattering.**
2026   [19586955] J R Soc Interface 6 Suppl 5(-):S611-7 (2009)

2009   **Bio-metals imaging and speciation in cells using proton and synchrotron radiation X-ray microspectroscopy.**
2027   [19605403] J R Soc Interface 6 Suppl 5(-):S649-58 (2009)

2006   **mda-7/IL-24: multifunctional cancer-specific apoptosis-inducing cytokine.**
2028   [16464504] Pharmacol Ther 111(3):596-628 (2006)

2011   **Mechanisms of termination and prevention of atrial fibrillation by drug therapy.**
2029   [21334377] Pharmacol Ther 131(2):221-41 (2011)

2011   **Transient receptor potential (TRP) channels as drug targets for diseases of the digestive system.**
2030   [21420431] Pharmacol Ther 131(1):142-70 (2011)

2011   **Targeting stem cell niches and trafficking for cardiovascular therapy.**
2031   [20965213] Pharmacol Ther 129(1):62-81 (2011)

2008   **Constitutive activation of G protein-coupled receptors and diseases: insights into mechanisms of activation and therapeutics.**
2032   [18768149] Pharmacol Ther 120(2):129-48 (2008)

2010   **A current view of brain renin-angiotensin system: Is the (pro)renin receptor the missing link?**
2033   [19723538] Pharmacol Ther 125(1):27-38 (2010)

2010   **Effects of tempol and redox-cycling nitroxides in models of oxidative stress.**
2034   [20153367] Pharmacol Ther 126(2):119-45 (2010)

2007   **R4 RGS proteins: regulation of G-protein signaling and beyond.**
2035   [18006065] Pharmacol Ther 116(3):473-95 (2007)

2007
2036

Small molecules affecting transcription in Friedreich ataxia.
[17826840] Pharmacol Ther 116(2):236-48 (2007)

2009
2037

Physiological and pharmacological implications of beta-arrestin regulation.
[19100766] Pharmacol Ther 121(3):285-93 (2009)

2007
2038

Mechanistic pathways and biological roles for receptor-independent activators of G-protein signaling.
[17240454] Pharmacol Ther 113(3):488-506 (2007)

2005
2039

Cellular mechanisms underlying acquired epilepsy: the calcium hypothesis of the induction and maintainance of epilepsy.
[15737406] Pharmacol Ther 105(3):229-66 (2005)

2009
2040

Ryanodine receptor-mediated arrhythmias and sudden cardiac death.
[19345240] Pharmacol Ther 123(2):151-77 (2009)

2009
2041

Adenosine signaling and the regulation of chronic lung disease.
[19426761] Pharmacol Ther 123(1):105-16 (2009)

2009
2042

30 years of dynorphins--new insights on their functions in neuropsychiatric diseases.
[19481570] Pharmacol Ther 123(3):353-70 (2009)

2009
2043

Cooperative properties of cytochromes P450.
[19555717] Pharmacol Ther 124(2):151-67 (2009)

2008
2044

Pharmacological approach to the treatment of long and short QT syndromes.
[18378319] Pharmacol Ther 118(1):138-51 (2008)

2009
2045

The pharmacology of sigma-1 receptors.
[19619582] Pharmacol Ther 124(2):195-206 (2009)

2006
2046

The structural basis of arrestin-mediated regulation of G-protein-coupled receptors.
[16460808] Pharmacol Ther 110(3):465-502 (2006)

2008
2047

The chemical neuroanatomy of breathing.
[18706532] Respir Physiol Neurobiol 164(1-2):3-11 (2008)

2004
2048

A unique pathway of cardiac myocyte death caused by hypoxia-acidosis.
[15299040] J Exp Biol 207(Pt 18):3189-200 (2004)

2003
2049

Chitin metabolism in insects: structure, function and regulation of chitin synthases and chitinases.
[14610026] J Exp Biol 206(Pt 24):4393-412 (2003)

2003
2050

Four-dimensional organization of protein kinase signaling cascades: the roles of diffusion, endocytosis and molecular motors.
[12756289] J Exp Biol 206(Pt 12):2073-82 (2003)

2010
2051

Epigenetics and transgenerational transfer: a physiological perspective.
[20008356] J Exp Biol 213(1):3-16 (2010)

2007
2052

Historical reconstructions of evolving physiological complexity: O2 secretion in the eye and swimbladder of fishes.
[17449830] J Exp Biol 210(Pt 9):1641-52 (2007)

2009
2053

Regulation of the V-ATPase in kidney epithelial cells: dual role in acid-base homeostasis and vesicle trafficking.
[19448085] J Exp Biol 212(Pt 11):1762-72 (2009)

2009
2054

The little we know on the structure and machinery of V-ATPase.
[19448070] J Exp Biol 212(Pt 11):1604-10 (2009)

2009   **Voltage coupling of primary H+ V-ATPases to secondary Na+- or K+-dependent transporters.**
2055   [19448072] J Exp Biol 212(Pt 11):1620-9 (2009)

2010   **Dynamic fluorescence depolarization: a powerful tool to explore protein folding on the ribosome.**
2056   [20685617] Methods 52(1):57-73 (2010)

2010   **Everything you wanted to know about Markov State Models but were afraid to ask.**
2057   [20570730] Methods 52(1):99-105 (2010)

2010   **Genomic SELEX: a discovery tool for genomic aptamers.**
2058   [20541015] Methods 52(2):125-32 (2010)

2010   **Direct physical study of kinetochore-microtubule interactions by reconstitution and interrogation with an optical force clamp.**
2059   [20096784] Methods 51(2):242-50 (2010)

2010   **Approaches toward super-resolution fluorescence imaging of mitochondrial proteins using PALM.**
2060   [20060907] Methods 51(4):458-63 (2010)

2006   **Analyzing chromatin remodeling complexes using shotgun proteomics and normalized spectral abundance factors.**
2061   [17101441] Methods 40(4):303-11 (2006)

2009   **Raman crystallography of RNA.**
2062   [19409996] Methods 49(2):101-11 (2009)

2009   **Exploring ribozyme conformational changes with X-ray crystallography.**
2063   [19559088] Methods 49(2):87-100 (2009)

2008   **Experimental validation of miRNA targets.**
2064   [18158132] Methods 44(1):47-54 (2008)

2008   **Identification of microRNAs and other small regulatory RNAs using cDNA library sequencing.**
2065   [18158127] Methods 44(1):3-12 (2008)

2008   **Chemical calcium indicators.**
2066   [18929663] Methods 46(3):143-51 (2008)

2008   **Bimolecular fluorescence complementation (BiFC) analysis of protein interactions in Caenorhabditis elegans.**
2067   [18586101] Methods 45(3):185-91 (2008)

2011   **The beating heart of melanomas: a minor subset of cancer cells sustains tumor growth.**
2068   [21487158] Oncotarget 2(4):313-20 (2011)

2010   **Epithelial mesenchymal transition and tumor budding in aggressive colorectal cancer: tumor budding as oncotarget.**
2069   [21317460] Oncotarget 1(7):651-61 (2010)

2010   **Genomic damage in endstage renal disease-contribution of uremic toxins.**
2070   [22069557] Toxins (Basel) 2(10):2340-58 (2010)

2008   **Optical switches for remote and noninvasive control of cell signaling.**
2071   [18927384] Science 322(5900):395-9 (2008)

2010   **O-GlcNAc signaling: a metabolic link between diabetes and cancer?**
2072   [20466550] Trends Biochem Sci 35(10):547-55 (2010)

2010   **The Sec14 superfamily and mechanisms for crosstalk between lipid metabolism and lipid signaling.**
2073   [19926291] Trends Biochem Sci 35(3):150-60 (2010)

2007   **Molecular biology of PCSK9: its role in LDL metabolism.**
2074   [17215125] Trends Biochem Sci 32(2):71-7 (2007)

2010   **GSK3: a multifaceted kinase in Wnt signaling.**
2075   [19884009] Trends Biochem Sci 35(3):161-8 (2010)

2010   **Yorkie: the final destination of Hippo signaling.**
2076   [20452772] Trends Cell Biol 20(7):410-7 (2010)

2010   **DNA methylation and cellular reprogramming.**
2077   [20810283] Trends Cell Biol 20(10):609-17 (2010)

2010   **NuMA after 30 years: the matrix revisited.**
2078   [20137953] Trends Cell Biol 20(4):214-22 (2010)

2008   **Using plasma membrane nanoclusters to build better signaling circuits.**
2079   [18620858] Trends Cell Biol 18(8):364-71 (2008)

2008   **Cytonemes and tunneling nanotubules in cell-cell communication and viral pathogenesis.**
2080   [18703335] Trends Cell Biol 18(9):414-20 (2008)

2009   **The 14-3-3 proteins: integrators of diverse signaling cues that impact cell fate and cancer development.**
2081   [19027299] Trends Cell Biol 19(1):16-23 (2009)

2010   **Intermediate filaments take the heat as stress proteins.**
2082   [20045331] Trends Cell Biol 20(2):79-91 (2010)

2007   **The Gli code: an information nexus regulating cell fate, stemness and cancer.**
2083   [17845852] Trends Cell Biol 17(9):438-47 (2007)

2009   **MAM: more than just a housekeeper.**
2084   [19144519] Trends Cell Biol 19(2):81-8 (2009)

2008   **Apoptosis-induced compensatory proliferation. The Cell is dead. Long live the Cell!**
2085   [18774295] Trends Cell Biol 18(10):467-73 (2008)

2009   **Imaging endocytic clathrin structures in living cells.**
2086   [19836955] Trends Cell Biol 19(11):596-605 (2009)

2009   **Polycomb group complexes--many combinations, many functions.**
2087   [19889541] Trends Cell Biol 19(12):692-704 (2009)

2010   **Nuclear phosphoinositides: a signaling enigma wrapped in a compartmental conundrum.**
2088   [19846310] Trends Cell Biol 20(1):25-35 (2010)

2009   **A single molecule view of gene expression.**
2089   [19819144] Trends Cell Biol 19(11):630-7 (2009)

2009   **Caught in the act: quantifying protein behaviour in living cells.**
2090   [19801189] Trends Cell Biol 19(11):566-74 (2009)

2005   **From the recent lessons of the Malagasy foci towards a global understanding of the factors involved in plague reemergence.**
2091   [15845233] Vet Res 36(3):437-53 (2005)

2010   **Virotherapy against malignant glioma stem cells.**
2092   [19643532] Cancer Lett 289(1):1-10 (2010)

| 2010 | **Purinergic mechanisms in breast cancer support intravasation, extravasation and angiogenesis.** |
| 2093 | [19926395] Cancer Lett 291(2):131-41 (2010) |

| 2010 | **Molecular mechanisms involved in farnesol-induced apoptosis.** |
| 2094 | [19520495] Cancer Lett 287(2):123-35 (2010) |

| 2007 | **Dysadherin: a new player in cancer progression.** |
| 2095 | [17442482] Cancer Lett 255(2):161-9 (2007) |

| 2009 | **Putative roles of hepatitis B x antigen in the pathogenesis of chronic liver disease.** |
| 2096 | [19201080] Cancer Lett 286(1):69-79 (2009) |

| 2009 | **Emerging role of Notch in stem cells and cancer.** |
| 2097 | [19022563] Cancer Lett 279(1):8-12 (2009) |

| 2009 | **Targeting tumor angiogenesis with histone deacetylase inhibitors.** |
| 2098 | [19111391] Cancer Lett 280(2):145-53 (2009) |

| 2008 | **Nitric oxide as a target of complementary and alternative medicines to prevent and treat inflammation and cancer.** |
| 2099 | [18440130] Cancer Lett 268(1):10-30 (2008) |

| 2008 | **Cancer chemotherapy with indole-3-carbinol, bis(3'-indolyl)methane and synthetic analogs.** |
| 2100 | [18501502] Cancer Lett 269(2):326-38 (2008) |

| 2010 | **Phage display in molecular imaging and diagnosis of cancer.** |
| 2101 | [20170129] Chem Rev 110(5):3196-211 (2010) |

| 2010 | **Mass spectrometric imaging for biomedical tissue analysis.** |
| 2102 | [20423155] Chem Rev 110(5):3237-77 (2010) |

| 2009 | **Modeling kinetics of subcellular disposition of chemicals.** |
| 2103 | [19265398] Chem Rev 109(5):1793-899 (2009) |

| 2009 | **Coherent multidimensional optical spectroscopy of excitons in molecular aggregates; quasiparticle versus supermolecule perspectives.** |
| 2104 | [19432416] Chem Rev 109(6):2350-408 (2009) |

| 2010 | **C-type lectins, fungi and Th17 responses.** |
| 2105 | [21075040] Cytokine Growth Factor Rev 21(6):405-12 (2010) |

| 2010 | **Transforming growth factor beta (TGF-beta) and inflammation in cancer.** |
| 2106 | [20018551] Cytokine Growth Factor Rev 21(1):49-59 (2010) |

| 2007 | **A scientific journey through the 2-5A/RNase L system.** |
| 2107 | [17681844] Cytokine Growth Factor Rev 18(5-6):381-8 (2007) |

| 2007 | **The response of mammalian cells to double-stranded RNA.** |
| 2108 | [17698400] Cytokine Growth Factor Rev 18(5-6):363-71 (2007) |

| 2008 | **IGF2: epigenetic regulation and role in development and disease.** |
| 2109 | [18308616] Cytokine Growth Factor Rev 19(2):111-20 (2008) |

| 2008 | **Crosstalk via the NF-kappaB signaling system.** |
| 2110 | [18515173] Cytokine Growth Factor Rev 19(3-4):187-97 (2008) |

| 2008 | **microRNAs and death receptors.** |
| 2111 | [18490189] Cytokine Growth Factor Rev 19(3-4):303-11 (2008) |

2009   **Control of microRNA biogenesis by TGFbeta signaling pathway-A novel role of Smads in the nucleus.**
2112   [19892582] Cytokine Growth Factor Rev 20(5-6):517-21 (2009)

2008   **Plasmacytoid dendritic cells and type I IFN: 50 years of convergent history.**
2113   [18248767] Cytokine Growth Factor Rev 19(1):3-19 (2008)

2008   **MALDI imaging mass spectrometry for direct tissue analysis: a new frontier for molecular histology.**
2114   [18618129] Histochem Cell Biol 130(3):421-34 (2008)

2008   **Morphological and cytochemical determination of cell death by apoptosis.**
2115   [18000678] Histochem Cell Biol 129(1):33-43 (2008)

2008   **The art of cellular communication: tunneling nanotubes bridge the divide.**
2116   [18386044] Histochem Cell Biol 129(5):539-50 (2008)

2008   **Actin: its cumbersome pilgrimage through cellular compartments.**
2117   [18438682] Histochem Cell Biol 129(6):695-704 (2008)

2008   **Structure and function of mammalian cilia.**
2118   [18365235] Histochem Cell Biol 129(6):687-93 (2008)

2008   **Tight junctions and the modulation of barrier function in disease.**
2119   [18415116] Histochem Cell Biol 130(1):55-70 (2008)

2008   **Autophagy-physiology and pathophysiology.**
2120   [18320203] Histochem Cell Biol 129(4):407-20 (2008)

2008   **Connexons and cell adhesion: a romantic phase.**
2121   [18481075] Histochem Cell Biol 130(1):71-7 (2008)

2008   **The renal cortical interstitium: morphological and functional aspects.**
2122   [18575881] Histochem Cell Biol 130(2):247-62 (2008)

2008   **Bridging fluorescence microscopy and electron microscopy.**
2123   [18575880] Histochem Cell Biol 130(2):211-7 (2008)

2008   **The epithelial cholinergic system of the airways.**
2124   [18566825] Histochem Cell Biol 130(2):219-34 (2008)

2008   **Imaging aspects of cardiovascular disease at the cell and molecular level.**
2125   [18506469] Histochem Cell Biol 130(2):235-45 (2008)

2008   **Genome-wide association studies: a new window into immune-mediated diseases.**
2126   [18654571] Nat Rev Immunol 8(8):631-43 (2008)

2008   **How regulatory T cells work.**
2127   [18566595] Nat Rev Immunol 8(7):523-32 (2008)

2008   **Interferon-inducible antiviral effectors.**
2128   [18575461] Nat Rev Immunol 8(7):559-68 (2008)

2004   **Fibrotic disease and the T(H)1/T(H)2 paradigm.**
2129   [15286725] Nat Rev Immunol 4(8):583-94 (2004)

2010   **Macrophage death and defective inflammation resolution in atherosclerosis.**
2130   [19960040] Nat Rev Immunol 10(1):36-46 (2010)

2008   **Transcriptional regulation by AIRE: molecular mechanisms of central tolerance.**
2131   [19008896] Nat Rev Immunol 8(12):948-57 (2008)

2009   **Myeloid-derived suppressor cells as regulators of the immune system.**
2132   [19197294] Nat Rev Immunol 9(3):162-74 (2009)

2009   **Immunogenic and tolerogenic cell death.**
2133   [19365408] Nat Rev Immunol 9(5):353-63 (2009)

2009   **Immunoregulatory functions of mTOR inhibition.**
2134   [19390566] Nat Rev Immunol 9(5):324-37 (2009)

2008   **How dying cells alert the immune system to danger.**
2135   [18340345] Nat Rev Immunol 8(4):279-89 (2008)

2008   **Cis interactions of immunoreceptors with MHC and non-MHC ligands.**
2136   [18309314] Nat Rev Immunol 8(4):269-78 (2008)

2008   **The alliance of sphingosine-1-phosphate and its receptors in immunity.**
2137   [18787560] Nat Rev Immunol 8(10):753-63 (2008)

2008   **Resolving inflammation: dual anti-inflammatory and pro-resolution lipid mediators.**
2138   [18437155] Nat Rev Immunol 8(5):349-61 (2008)

2009   **Stromal cell contributions to the homeostasis and functionality of the immune system.**
2139   [19644499] Nat Rev Immunol 9(9):618-29 (2009)

2011   **Role of microRNAs in endothelial cell pathophysiology.**
2140   [21946298] Pol Arch Med Wewn 121(10):361-6 (2011)

2010   **Management of dyspnea in patients with advanced lung or heart disease: practical guidance from the American college of chest physicians consensus statement.**
2141   [20502400] Pol Arch Med Wewn 120(5):160-6 (2010)

2002   **Assumptions of the tumor 'escape' hypothesis.**
2142   [11926416] Semin Cancer Biol 12(1):81-6 (2002)

2009   **Hexokinase-2 bound to mitochondria: cancer's stygian link to the "Warburg Effect" and a pivotal target for effective therapy.**
2143   [19101634] Semin Cancer Biol 19(1):17-24 (2009)

2009   **Is Akt the "Warburg kinase"?-Akt-energy metabolism interactions and oncogenesis.**
2144   [19130886] Semin Cancer Biol 19(1):25-31 (2009)

2007   **Tumor immunoediting and immunosculpting pathways to cancer progression.**
2145   [17662614] Semin Cancer Biol 17(4):275-87 (2007)

2007   **MicroRNAs and genomic instability.**
2146   [17113784] Semin Cancer Biol 17(1):65-73 (2007)

2008   **Theories of carcinogenesis: an emerging perspective.**
2147   [18472276] Semin Cancer Biol 18(5):372-7 (2008)

2006   **Myc in model organisms: a view from the flyroom.**
2148   [16916612] Semin Cancer Biol 16(4):303-12 (2006)

2008   **HIV-associated nephropathy: clinical presentation, pathology, and epidemiology in the era of antiretroviral therapy.**
2149   [19013322] Semin Nephrol 28(6):513-22 (2008)

2007   **Direct tissue analysis by matrix-assisted laser desorption ionization mass spectrometry: application to kidney biology.**
2150   [18061842] Semin Nephrol 27(6):597-608 (2007)

2007   **Histopathology of diabetic nephropathy.**
2151   [17418688] Semin Nephrol 27(2):195-207 (2007)

2009   **The physiology of urinary concentration: an update.**
2152   [19523568] Semin Nephrol 29(3):178-95 (2009)

2008   **Role of interstitial apatite plaque in the pathogenesis of the common calcium oxalate stone.**
2153   [18359392] Semin Nephrol 28(2):111-9 (2008)

2008   **The future of pediatric acute kidney injury management--biomarkers.**
2154   [18790370] Semin Nephrol 28(5):493-8 (2008)

2008   **Vasopressin and aquaporin 2 in clinical disorders of water homeostasis.**
2155   [18519089] Semin Nephrol 28(3):289-96 (2008)

2008   **Bypassing vasopressin receptor signaling pathways in nephrogenic diabetes insipidus.**
2156   [18519087] Semin Nephrol 28(3):266-78 (2008)

2008   **Dissecting the roles of aquaporins in renal pathophysiology using transgenic mice.**
2157   [18519083] Semin Nephrol 28(3):217-26 (2008)

2009   **Podocytes and glomerular function with aging.**
2158   [20006790] Semin Nephrol 29(6):587-93 (2009)

2009   **Cell and molecular biology of kidney development.**
2159   [19615554] Semin Nephrol 29(4):321-37 (2009)

2007   **Quest for the basic plan of nervous system circuitry.**
2160   [17267046] Brain Res Rev 55(2):356-72 (2007)

2007   **The radial edifice of cortical architecture: from neuronal silhouettes to genetic engineering.**
2161   [17467805] Brain Res Rev 55(2):204-19 (2007)

2007   **Neural networks a century after Cajal.**
2162   [17692925] Brain Res Rev 55(2):264-84 (2007)

2007   **Phosphene induction by microstimulation of macaque V1.**
2163   [17173976] Brain Res Rev 53(2):337-43 (2007)

2009   **The neuroprotective properties of calorie restriction, the ketogenic diet, and ketone bodies.**
2164   [18845187] Brain Res Rev 59(2):293-315 (2009)

2009   **Autism, fever, epigenetics and the locus coeruleus.**
2165   [19059284] Brain Res Rev 59(2):388-92 (2009)

2007   **Neuroimmunopathology in a murine model of neuropsychiatric lupus.**
2166   [17223198] Brain Res Rev 54(1):67-79 (2007)

2008   **Endogenous and synthetic neurosteroids in treatment of Niemann-Pick Type C disease.**
2167   [17629950] Brain Res Rev 57(2):410-20 (2008)

2008   **Behavioral characteristics and neurobiological substrates shared by Pavlovian sign-tracking and drug abuse.**
2168   [18234349] Brain Res Rev 58(1):121-35 (2008)

2010   **JAB1/CSN5: a new player in cell cycle control and cancer.**
2169   [20955608] Cell Div 5(-):26 (2010)

2010   **Merotelic attachments and non-homologous end joining are the basis of chromosomal instability.**
2170   [20478024] Cell Div 5(-):13 (2010)

2010
2171

An overview of Cdk1-controlled targets and processes.
[20465793] Cell Div 5(-):11 (2010)

2010
2172

Role of senescence and mitotic catastrophe in cancer therapy.
[20205872] Cell Div 5(-):4 (2010)

2007
2173

Stealing the spotlight: CUL4-DDB1 ubiquitin ligase docks WD40-repeat proteins to destroy.
[17280619] Cell Div 2(-):5 (2007)

2007
2174

Irreversibility of cellular senescence: dual roles of p16INK4a/Rb-pathway in cell cycle control.
[17343761] Cell Div 2(-):10 (2007)

2007
2175

Resolving RAD51C function in late stages of homologous recombination.
[17547768] Cell Div 2(-):15 (2007)

2009
2176

Septins: molecular partitioning and the generation of cellular asymmetry.
[19709431] Cell Div 4(-):18 (2009)

2008
2177

The chromosomal passenger complex and the spindle assembly checkpoint: kinetochore-microtubule error correction and beyond.
[18507820] Cell Div 3(-):10 (2008)

2009
2178

Smurf2 as a novel mitotic regulator: From the spindle assembly checkpoint to tumorigenesis.
[19583833] Cell Div 4(-):14 (2009)

2010
2179

Imaging of inflammation by PET, conventional scintigraphy, and other imaging techniques.
[21078798] J Nucl Med 51(12):1937-49 (2010)

2010
2180

In vivo imaging of RNA interference.
[20080892] J Nucl Med 51(2):169-72 (2010)

2010
2181

Models of carcinogenesis: an overview.
[20430846] Carcinogenesis 31(10):1703-9 (2010)

2010
2182

Basic properties and molecular mechanisms of exogenous chemical carcinogens.
[19858070] Carcinogenesis 31(2):135-48 (2010)

2009
2183

Metabolic transformation in cancer.
[19321800] Carcinogenesis 30(8):1269-80 (2009)

2010
2184

Senescence: an antiviral defense that is tumor suppressive?
[19887513] Carcinogenesis 31(1):19-26 (2010)

2010
2185

Chemical biology of mutagenesis and DNA repair: cellular responses to DNA alkylation.
[19875697] Carcinogenesis 31(1):59-70 (2010)

2009
2186

Role of TRPV1 in inflammation-induced airway hypersensitivity.
[19269247] Curr Opin Pharmacol 9(3):243-9 (2009)

2009
2187

SSRIs act as selective brain steroidogenic stimulants (SBSSs) at low doses that are inactive on 5-HT reuptake.
[19157982] Curr Opin Pharmacol 9(1):24-30 (2009)

2008
2188

Drugs acting on SUR1 to treat CNS ischemia and trauma.
[18032110] Curr Opin Pharmacol 8(1):42-9 (2008)

2004
2189

Endocrine disruption by cadmium, a common environmental toxicant with paradoxical effects on reproduction.
[15096650] Exp Biol Med (Maywood) 229(5):383-92 (2004)

2009
2190
Cardiovascular applications of hyperpolarized contrast media and metabolic tracers.
[19934362] Exp Biol Med (Maywood) 234(12):1395-416 (2009)

2009
2191
Regulation of epithelial-mesenchymal transition in palatal fusion.
[19234053] Exp Biol Med (Maywood) 234(5):483-91 (2009)

2009
2192
Molecular targets of nutraceuticals derived from dietary spices: potential role in suppression of inflammation and tumorigenesis.
[19491364] Exp Biol Med (Maywood) 234(8):825-49 (2009)

2009
2193
Adiponectin: a key adipokine in alcoholic fatty liver.
[19491377] Exp Biol Med (Maywood) 234(8):850-9 (2009)

2009
2194
Mitochondrial nitric oxide synthase: a masterpiece of metabolic adaptation, cell growth, transformation, and death.
[19546350] Exp Biol Med (Maywood) 234(9):1020-8 (2009)

2008
2195
Alternate hypothesis on the pathogenesis of dengue hemorrhagic fever (DHF)/dengue shock syndrome (DSS) in dengue virus infection.
[18367628] Exp Biol Med (Maywood) 233(4):401-8 (2008)

2010
2196
Molecular mechanisms of adrenergic stimulation in the heart.
[20156590] Heart Rhythm 7(8):1151-3 (2010)

2010
2197
J wave syndromes.
[20153265] Heart Rhythm 7(4):549-58 (2010)

2009
2198
Basis for sudden cardiac death prediction by T-wave alternans from an integrative physiology perspective.
[19251221] Heart Rhythm 6(3):416-22 (2009)

2009
2199
Explaining the clinical manifestations of T wave alternans in patients at risk for sudden cardiac death.
[19168395] Heart Rhythm 6(3 Suppl):S22-8 (2009)

2007
2200
Triggered activity and atrial fibrillation.
[17336878] Heart Rhythm 4(3 Suppl):S17-23 (2007)

2007
2201
Autonomic nerves in pulmonary veins.
[17336886] Heart Rhythm 4(3 Suppl):S57-60 (2007)

2009
2202
The surgical treatment of atrial fibrillation.
[19631907] Heart Rhythm 6(8 Suppl):S45-50 (2009)

2008
2203
Magnetocardiography for fetal arrhythmias.
[18486565] Heart Rhythm 5(7):1073-6 (2008)

2009
2204
Drugs and Brugada syndrome patients: review of the literature, recommendations, and an up-to-date website (www.brugadadrugs.org).
[19716089] Heart Rhythm 6(9):1335-41 (2009)

2011
2205
Precursor cell biology and the development of astrocyte transplantation therapies: lessons from spinal cord injury.
[21918888] Neurotherapeutics 8(4):677-93 (2011)

2010
2206
Functions of astrocytes and their potential as therapeutic targets.
[20880499] Neurotherapeutics 7(4):338-53 (2010)

2010
2207
Astrocyte glutamine synthetase: importance in hyperammonemic syndromes and potential target for therapy.
[20880508] Neurotherapeutics 7(4):452-70 (2010)

2010
2208
Reactive astrocytes as therapeutic targets for CNS disorders.
[20880511] Neurotherapeutics 7(4):494-506 (2010)

2009
2209
Engineered adenosine-releasing cells for epilepsy therapy: human mesenchymal stem cells and human embryonic stem cells.
[19332320] Neurotherapeutics 6(2):278-83 (2009)

2003
2210
Brain reorganization after stroke.
[14681816] Top Stroke Rehabil 10(3):1-20 (2003)

2009
2211
The Bobath concept in contemporary clinical practice.
[19443348] Top Stroke Rehabil 16(1):57-68 (2009)

2008
2212
Brain-mapping techniques for evaluating poststroke recovery and rehabilitation: a review.
[19008203] Top Stroke Rehabil 15(5):427-50 (2008)

2010
2213
Mechanisms of neutrophil accumulation in the lungs against bacteria.
[19738160] Am J Respir Cell Mol Biol 43(1):5-16 (2010)

2004
2214
Molecular mechanisms of pulmonary peptidomimetic drug and peptide transport.
[14969997] Am J Respir Cell Mol Biol 30(3):251-60 (2004)

2008
2215
Alveolar epithelial beta2-adrenergic receptors.
[17709598] Am J Respir Cell Mol Biol 38(2):127-34 (2008)

2011
2216
The role of nebivolol in the prevention of contrast-induced nephropathy.
[21959876] Anadolu Kardiyol Derg 11(7):618 (2011)

2010
2217
High-throughput experimental studies to identify miRNA targets directly, with special focus on the mammalian brain.
[20380813] Brain Res 1338(-):122-30 (2010)

2010
2218
Role of the medial prefrontal cortex in coping and resilience.
[20727864] Brain Res 1355(-):52-60 (2010)

2010
2219
Lateral hypothalamic orexin/hypocretin neurons: A role in reward-seeking and addiction.
[19815001] Brain Res 1314(-):74-90 (2010)

2010
2220
A tiny touch: activation of cell signaling pathways with magnetic nanoparticles.
[20016028] Endocrinology 151(2):451-7 (2010)

2010
2221
Minireview: transgenerational inheritance of the stress response: a new frontier in stress research.
[19887563] Endocrinology 151(1):7-13 (2010)

2007
????
Targeting the Wnt/beta-catenin pathway to regulate bone formation in the adult skeleton.
[17395698] Endocrinology 148(6):2635-43 (2007)

2007
2223
In vivo analysis of Wnt signaling in bone.
[17395705] Endocrinology 148(6):2630-4 (2007)

2009
2224
Epigenetic alterations in human prostate cancers.
[19520778] Endocrinology 150(9):3991-4002 (2009)

2005
2225
Minireview: hexose-6-phosphate dehydrogenase and redox control of 11{beta}-hydroxysteroid dehydrogenase type 1 activity.
[15774558] Endocrinology 146(6):2539-43 (2005)

2009
2226
Severe preeclampsia-related changes in gene expression at the maternal-fetal interface include sialic acid-binding immunoglobulin-like lectin-6 and pappalysin-2.
[18818296] Endocrinology 150(1):452-62 (2009)

2011   **Lorcaserin: drug profile and illustrative model of the regulatory challenges of weight-loss drug**
2227   **development.**
[21438803] Expert Rev Cardiovasc Ther 9(3):265-77 (2011)

2010   **Systematic review of reversible cerebral vasoconstriction syndrome.**
2228   [20936928] Expert Rev Cardiovasc Ther 8(10):1417-21 (2010)

2009   **Treatment of combined hypertension and orthostatic hypotension in older adults: more questions**
2229   **than answers still remain.**
[19505268] Expert Rev Cardiovasc Ther 7(6):557-60 (2009)

2008   **A review of known imprinting syndromes and their association with assisted reproduction**
2230   **technologies.**
[18703582] Hum Reprod 23(12):2826-34 (2008)

2004   **The peptide nucleic acids: a new way for chromosomal investigation on isolated cells?**
2231   [15229198] Hum Reprod 19(9):1946-51 (2004)

2007   **Tubal ectopic pregnancy: macrophages under the microscope.**
2232   [17664241] Hum Reprod 22(10):2577-84 (2007)

2006   **Intrauterine insemination catheters for assisted reproduction: a systematic review and meta-analysis.**
2233   [16675484] Hum Reprod 21(8):1961-7 (2006)

2010   **Dynamic organization of lymphocyte plasma membrane: lessons from advanced imaging methods.**
2234   [20646076] Immunology 131(1):1-8 (2010)

2010   **Immunoinformatics: an integrated scenario.**
2235   [20722763] Immunology 131(2):153-68 (2010)

2010   **T-cell receptor revision: friend or foe?**
2236   [20201984] Immunology 129(4):467-73 (2010)

2008   **Neutrophil mobilization and clearance in the bone marrow.**
2237   [19128361] Immunology 125(3):281-8 (2008)

2010   **The extensive polymorphism of KIR genes.**
2238   [20028428] Immunology 129(1):8-19 (2010)

2010   **T-cell exhaustion: characteristics, causes and conversion.**
2239   [20201977] Immunology 129(4):474-81 (2010)

2009   **Epigenetics and T helper 1 differentiation.**
2240   [19178593] Immunology 126(3):299-305 (2009)

2009   **Regulation of different inflammatory diseases by impacting the mevalonate pathway.**
2241   [19191903] Immunology 127(1):18-25 (2009)

2009   **Following TRAIL's path in the immune system.**
2242   [19476510] Immunology 127(2):145-54 (2009)

2009   **Endosomal processing for antigen presentation mediated by CD1 and Class I major**
2243   **histocompatibility complex: roads to display or destruction.**
[19476512] Immunology 127(2):163-70 (2009)

2009   **An integrated view of the regulation of NKG2D ligands.**
2244   [19689730] Immunology 128(1):1-6 (2009)

2011   **Novel approaches to in vitro transgenesis.**
2245   [21134989] J Endocrinol 208(3):193-206 (2011)

2011
2246
The mislabelling of deoxycorticosterone: making sense of corticosteroid structure and function.
[21715433] J Endocrinol 211(1):3-16 (2011)

2008
2247
Epithelial injury induces an innate repair mechanism linked to cellular senescence and fibrosis involving IGF-binding protein-5.
[18676497] J Endocrinol 199(2):155-64 (2008)

2010
2248
Mechanisms behind the non-thyroidal illness syndrome: an update.
[20016054] J Endocrinol 205(1):1-13 (2010)

2007
2249
Circadian clocks: regulators of endocrine and metabolic rhythms.
[17951531] J Endocrinol 195(2):187-98 (2007)

2009
2250
Sprouty proteins: modified modulators, matchmakers or missing links?
[19423641] J Endocrinol 203(2):191-202 (2009)

2005
2251
11beta-hydroxysteroid dehydrogenase and the pre-receptor regulation of corticosteroid hormone action.
[16079253] J Endocrinol 186(2):251-71 (2005)

2011
2252
Diastolic myofilament dysfunction in the failing human heart.
[21487693] Pflugers Arch 462(1):155-63 (2011)

2011
2253
Assessment of contractility in intact ventricular cardiomyocytes using the dimensionless 'Frank-Starling Gain' index.
[21494804] Pflugers Arch 462(1):39-48 (2011)

2009
2254
Micropuncturing the nephron.
[18752000] Pflugers Arch 458(1):189-201 (2009)

2008
2255
The non-excitable smooth muscle: calcium signaling and phenotypic switching during vascular disease.
[18365243] Pflugers Arch 456(5):769-85 (2008)

2008
2256
New developments in the signaling mechanisms of the store-operated calcium entry pathway.
[18536932] Pflugers Arch 457(2):405-15 (2008)

2008
2257
Renal function and mitochondrial cytopathy (MC): more questions than answers?
[18487272] QJM 101(10):755-66 (2008)

2004
2258
Thoracoscopic management of thoracic duct injury: Is there a place for conservatism?
[15048002] J Postgrad Med 50(1):57-9 (2004)

2003
2259
The glucose paradox of cerebral ischaemia.
[14699225] J Postgrad Med 49(4):299-301 (2003)

2007
2260
Human aldo-keto reductases: Function, gene regulation, and single nucleotide polymorphisms.
[17537398] Arch Biochem Biophys 464(2):241-50 (2007)

2008
2261
The chemistry of cell signaling by reactive oxygen and nitrogen species and 4-hydroxynonenal.
[18602883] Arch Biochem Biophys 477(2):183-95 (2008)

2010
2262
New role for plasmin in sodium homeostasis.
[19864949] Curr Opin Nephrol Hypertens 19(1):13-9 (2010)

2009
2263
Vascular signaling through G protein-coupled receptors: new concepts.
[19434053] Curr Opin Nephrol Hypertens 18(2):153-9 (2009)

2009
2264
Update on the glomerular filtration barrier.
[19374010] Curr Opin Nephrol Hypertens 18(3):226-32 (2009)

2008
2265

Epithelial junctions and polarity: complexes and kinases.
[18695392] Curr Opin Nephrol Hypertens 17(5):506-12 (2008)

2008
2266

Do thiazides worsen metabolic syndrome and renal disease? The pivotal roles for hyperuricemia and hypokalemia.
[18695387] Curr Opin Nephrol Hypertens 17(5):470-6 (2008)

2009
2267

The physiological impact of the serum and glucocorticoid-inducible kinase SGK1.
[19584721] Curr Opin Nephrol Hypertens 18(5):439-48 (2009)

2009
2268

Complications related to endoscopic retrograde cholangiopancreatography: a comprehensive clinical review.
[19337638] J Gastrointestin Liver Dis 18(1):73-82 (2009)

2008
2269

Confocal endomicroscopy for in vivo microscopic analysis of upper gastrointestinal tract premalignant and malignant lesions.
[18392254] J Gastrointestin Liver Dis 17(1):95-100 (2008)

2010
2270

Matricryptic sites control tissue injury responses in the cardiovascular system: relationships to pattern recognition receptor regulated events.
[19751741] J Mol Cell Cardiol 48(3):454-60 (2010)

2010
2271

Cardiac extracellular matrix remodeling: fibrillar collagens and Secreted Protein Acidic and Rich in Cysteine (SPARC).
[19577572] J Mol Cell Cardiol 48(3):544-9 (2010)

2009
2272

Cistromics of hormone-dependent cancer.
[19369485] Endocr Relat Cancer 16(2):381-9 (2009)

2009
2273

Mouse models of altered protein kinase A signaling.
[19470615] Endocr Relat Cancer 16(3):773-93 (2009)

2008
2274

Pituitary tumor-transforming gene in endocrine and other neoplasms: a review and update.
[18753362] Endocr Relat Cancer 15(3):721-43 (2008)

2004
2275

Bichat guidelines for the clinical management of haemorrhagic fever viruses and bioterrorism-related haemorrhagic fever viruses.
[15677844] Euro Surveill 9(12):E11-2 (2004)

2006
2276

Connecting thalamus and cortex: the role of ephrins.
[16411249] Anat Rec A Discov Mol Cell Evol Biol 288(2):135-42 (2006)

2006
2277

Evolutionary changes in the cochlea and labyrinth: Solving the problem of sound transmission to the balance organs of the inner ear.
[16552774] Anat Rec A Discov Mol Cell Evol Biol 288(4):482-9 (2006)

2004
2278

Hemangioblasts, angioblasts, and adult endothelial cell progenitors.
[14699630] Anat Rec A Discov Mol Cell Evol Biol 276(1):13-21 (2004)

2004
2279

Neuroregulation of the neuroendocrine compartment of the liver.
[15382010] Anat Rec A Discov Mol Cell Evol Biol 280(1):910-23 (2004)

2004
2280

Neural regulation of the hepatic circadian rhythm.
[15382011] Anat Rec A Discov Mol Cell Evol Biol 280(1):901-9 (2004)

2004
2281

Neural control of hepatic osmolytes and parenchymal cell hydration.
[15382012] Anat Rec A Discov Mol Cell Evol Biol 280(1):893-900 (2004)

2004
2282

Control of hepatocyte metabolism by sympathetic and parasympathetic hepatic nerves.
[15382015] Anat Rec A Discov Mol Cell Evol Biol 280(1):854-67 (2004)

2004
2283
Anatomy of efferent hepatic nerves.
[15382019] Anat Rec A Discov Mol Cell Evol Biol 280(1):821-6 (2004)

2004
2284
Neural connections between the hypothalamus and the liver.
[15382020] Anat Rec A Discov Mol Cell Evol Biol 280(1):808-20 (2004)

2004
2285
Cytoarchitecture and intercalated disks of the working myocardium and the conduction system in the mammalian heart.
[15368339] Anat Rec A Discov Mol Cell Evol Biol 280(2):940-51 (2004)

2004
2286
Structure-function relationship in the AV junction.
[15368340] Anat Rec A Discov Mol Cell Evol Biol 280(2):952-65 (2004)

2004
2287
Nature, significance, and mechanisms of electrical heterogeneities in ventricle.
[15368342] Anat Rec A Discov Mol Cell Evol Biol 280(2):1010-7 (2004)

2004
2288
Autoimmune-associated congenital heart block: dissecting the cascade from immunologic insult to relentless fibrosis.
[15368347] Anat Rec A Discov Mol Cell Evol Biol 280(2):1027-35 (2004)

2003
2289
Functional morphology of pulmonary neuroepithelial bodies: extremely complex airway receptors.
[12494487] Anat Rec A Discov Mol Cell Evol Biol 270(1):25-40 (2003)

2003
2290
Friedrich Sigmund Merkel and his "Merkel cell", morphology, development, and physiology: review and new results.
[12552639] Anat Rec A Discov Mol Cell Evol Biol 271(1):225-39 (2003)

2007
2291
Neurological disorders presenting mainly in adolescence.
[17264287] Arch Dis Child 92(2):170-5 (2007)

2010
2292
Antivascular effects of electrochemotherapy: implications in treatment of bleeding metastases.
[20470005] Expert Rev Anticancer Ther 10(5):729-46 (2010)

2009
2293
HuR modulates gemcitabine efficacy: new perspectives in pancreatic cancer treatment.
[19828005] Expert Rev Anticancer Ther 9(10):1439-41 (2009)

2011
2294
Adenovirus-mediated intratumoral expression of immunostimulatory proteins in combination with systemic Treg inactivation induces tumor-destructive immune responses in mouse models.
[21394107] Cancer Gene Ther 18(6):407-18 (2011)

2004
2295
Modulation of gene expression in human central nervous system tumors under methionine deprivation-induced stress.
[15492278] Cancer Res 64(20):7513-25 (2004)

2011
2296
Naturally occurring, tumor-specific, therapeutic proteins.
[21521711] Exp Biol Med (Maywood) 236(5):524-36 (2011)

2006
2297
Mitotic arrest, apoptosis, and sensitization to chemotherapy of melanomas by methionine deprivation stress.
[16908595] Mol Cancer Res 4(8):575-89 (2006)

2010
2298
Melanoma differentiation associated gene-7/interleukin-24 potently induces apoptosis in human myeloid leukemia cells through a process regulated by endoplasmic reticulum stress.
[20858700] Mol Pharmacol 78(6):1096-104 (2010)

2010
2299
Eradication of therapy-resistant human prostate tumors using an ultrasound-guided site-specific cancer terminator virus delivery approach.
[19888195] Mol Ther 18(2):295-306 (2010)

2010
2300
The development of MDA-7/IL-24 as a cancer therapeutic.
[20732354] Pharmacol Ther 128(2):375-84 (2010)

2012
2301
MDA-7/IL-24 Induces Bcl-2 Denitrosylation and Ubiquitin-Degradation Involved in Cancer Cell Apoptosis.
[22629368] PLoS One 7(5):e37200 (2012)

2009
2302
New microbicidal functions of tracheal glands: defective anti-infectious response to Pseudomonas aeruginosa in cystic fibrosis.
[19399182] PLoS One 4(4):e5357 (2009)

2008
2303
Autocrine regulation of mda-7/IL-24 mediates cancer-specific apoptosis.
[18599461] Proc Natl Acad Sci U S A 105(28):9763-8 (2008)

2005
2304
Targeting gene expression selectively in cancer cells by using the progression-elevated gene-3 promoter.
[15647352] Proc Natl Acad Sci U S A 102(4):1059-64 (2005)

2009
2305
Induction of cytokine gene expression in human thyroid epithelial cells irradiated with HZE particles (iron ions).
[19772464] Radiat Res 172(4):437-43 (2009)

2010
2306
Making sense of G-quadruplex and i-motif functions in oncogene promoters.
[20670278] FEBS J 277(17):3459-69 (2010)

2010
2307
G-quadruplex nucleic acids and human disease.
[20670277] FEBS J 277(17):3470-88 (2010)

2005
2308
Protein families and RNA recognition.
[15853794] FEBS J 272(9):2088-97 (2005)

2005
2309
Examining multiprotein signaling complexes from all angles.
[16262684] FEBS J 272(21):5426-35 (2005)

2011
2310
Using the Delphi technique to determine which outcomes to measure in clinical trials: recommendations for the future based on a systematic review of existing studies.
[21283604] PLoS Med 8(1):e1000393 (2011)

2004
2311
An inflammatory cascade leading to hyperresistinemia in humans.
[15578112] PLoS Med 1(2):e45 (2004)

2009
2312
Systematic reviews of genetic association studies. Human Genome Epidemiology Network.
[19260758] PLoS Med 6(3):e28 (2009)

2009
2313
The unintended consequences of clinical trials regulations.
[19918557] PLoS Med 3(11):e1000131 (2009)

2010
2314
Detection of nitric oxide by electron paramagnetic resonance spectroscopy.
[20304044] Free Radic Biol Med 49(2):122-9 (2010)

2011
2315
Redox signaling in cardiac myocytes.
[21236334] Free Radic Biol Med 50(7):777-93 (2011)

2009
2316
Cytochrome c/cardiolipin relations in mitochondria: a kiss of death.
[19285551] Free Radic Biol Med 46(11):1439-53 (2009)

2007
2317
Hyperoxia-induced signal transduction pathways in pulmonary epithelial cells.
[17349918] Free Radic Biol Med 42(7):897-908 (2007)

2009
2318
Convergence of nitric oxide and lipid signaling: anti-inflammatory nitro-fatty acids.
[19200454] Free Radic Biol Med 46(8):989-1003 (2009)

2009
2319
Heme oxygenase-1, a critical arbitrator of cell death pathways in lung injury and disease.
[19362144] Free Radic Biol Med 47(1):1-12 (2009)

2009 — Nrf2:INrf2 (Keap1) signaling in oxidative stress.
2320 — [19666107] Free Radic Biol Med 47(9):1304-9 (2009)

2008 — Nonequilibrium thermodynamics of thiol/disulfide redox systems: a perspective on redox systems biology.
2321 — [18155672] Free Radic Biol Med 44(6):921-37 (2008)

2008 — Endothelial cell regulation by phospholipid oxidation products.
2322 — [18460347] Free Radic Biol Med 45(2):119-23 (2008)

2008 — The chemical biology of nitric oxide: implications in cellular signaling.
2323 — [18439435] Free Radic Biol Med 45(1):18-31 (2008)

2008 — Redox-based regulation of signal transduction: principles, pitfalls, and promises.
2324 — [18423411] Free Radic Biol Med 45(1):1-17 (2008)

2009 — Tetrahydrobiopterin, superoxide, and vascular dysfunction.
2325 — [19628033] Free Radic Biol Med 47(8):1108-19 (2009)

2011 — Hepatitis associated aplastic anemia: a review.
2326 — [21352606] Virol J 8(-):87 (2011)

2011 — Cross-talk between cd1d-restricted nkt cells and Î³Î´ cells in t regulatory cell response.
2327 — [21255407] Virol J 8(-):32 (2011)

2007 — The PB1-F2 protein of Influenza A virus: increasing pathogenicity by disrupting alveolar macrophages.
2328 — [17224071] Virol J 4(-):9 (2007)

2010 — Drug- and non-drug-associated QT interval prolongation.
2329 — [20642543] Br J Clin Pharmacol 70(1):16-23 (2010)

2003 — Nitrate tolerance and the links with endothelial dysfunction and oxidative stress.
2330 — [14616421] Br J Clin Pharmacol 56(6):620-8 (2003)

2008 — Hormesis and medicine.
2331 — [18662293] Br J Clin Pharmacol 66(5):594-617 (2008)

2006 — Drugs for sleep disorders: mechanisms and therapeutic prospects.
2332 — [16722842] Br J Clin Pharmacol 61(6):761-6 (2006)

2011 — Significance testing as perverse probabilistic reasoning.
2333 — [21356064] BMC Med 9(-):20 (2011)

2011 — Regulation of vascular tone by adipocytes.
2334 — [21410966] BMC Med 9(-):25 (2011)

2011 — Enhancer of zeste homolog 2 (EZH2) in pediatric soft tissue sarcomas: first implications.
2335 — [21609503] BMC Med 9(-):63 (2011)

2009 — Disease-specific biomarker discovery by aptamers.
2336 — [19565638] Cytometry A 75(9):727-33 (2009)

2006 — Increasing lanthanide luminescence by use of the RETEL effect.
2337 — [16969811] Cytometry A 69(8):940-6 (2006)

2011 — Development of oral immunomodulatory agents in the management of multiple sclerosis.
2338 — [21625416] Drug Des Devel Ther 5(-):255-74 (2011)

2011
2339
Comparative assessment of biologics in treatment of psoriasis: drug design and clinical effectiveness of ustekinumab.
[21267358] Drug Des Devel Ther 5(-):41-9 (2011)

2011
2340
Ten simple rules for providing a scientific Web resource.
[21637800] PLoS Comput Biol 7(5):e1001126 (2011)

2005
2341
Quasispecies made simple.
[16322763] PLoS Comput Biol 1(6):e61 (2005)

2007
2342
Ten simple rules for a good poster presentation.
[17530921] PLoS Comput Biol 3(5):e102 (2007)

2007
2343
A primer on learning in Bayesian networks for computational biology.
[17784779] PLoS Comput Biol 3(8):e129 (2007)

2007
2344
The long and thorny road to publication in quality journals.
[18166071] PLoS Comput Biol 3(12):e251 (2007)

2008
2345
Defrosting the digital library: bibliographic tools for the next generation web.
[18974831] PLoS Comput Biol 4(10):e1000204 (2008)

2009
2346
What is stochastic resonance? Definitions, misconceptions, debates, and its relevance to biology.
[19562010] PLoS Comput Biol 5(5):e1000348 (2009)

2008
2347
Support vector machines and kernels for computational biology.
[18974822] PLoS Comput Biol 4(10):e1000173 (2008)

2007
2348
A review of feature selection techniques in bioinformatics.
[17720704] Bioinformatics 23(19):2507-17 (2007)

2007
2349
SNPchip: R classes and methods for SNP array data.
[17204461] Bioinformatics 23(5):627-8 (2007)

2005
2350
Co-occurrence based meta-analysis of scientific texts: retrieving biological relationships between genes.
[15657104] Bioinformatics 21(9):2049-58 (2005)

2009
2351
Schizophrenia susceptibility genes directly implicated in the life cycles of pathogens: cytomegalovirus, influenza, herpes simplex, rubella, and Toxoplasma gondii.
[18552348] Schizophr Bull 35(6):1163-82 (2009)

2010
2352
Hepatitis C virus hijacks host lipid metabolism.
[19854061] Trends Endocrinol Metab 21(1):33-40 (2010)

2010
2353
Epigenetic transgenerational actions of environmental factors in disease etiology.
[20074974] Trends Endocrinol Metab 21(4):214-22 (2010)

2009
2354
Nampt: linking NAD biology, metabolism and cancer.
[19109034] Trends Endocrinol Metab 20(3):130-8 (2009)

2009
2355
Torpor induction in mammals: recent discoveries fueling new ideas.
[19864159] Trends Endocrinol Metab 20(10):490-8 (2009)

2008
2356
New techniques for assessing arterial stiffness.
[18358423] Diabetes Metab 34 Suppl 1(-):S21-6 (2008)

2010
2357
RNA-targeted splice-correction therapy for neuromuscular disease.
[20150322] Brain 133(Pt 4):957-72 (2010)

2009
2358
The subependymal zone neurogenic niche: a beating heart in the centre of the brain: how plastic is adult neurogenesis? Opportunities for therapy and questions to be addressed.
[19773354] Brain 132(Pt 11):2909-21 (2009)

2004
2359
Methods to find out the expression of activated genes.
[15385048] Reprod Biol Endocrinol 2(-):68 (2004)

2010
2360
Information processing without brains--the power of intercellular regulators in plants.
[20332147] Development 137(8):1215-26 (2010)

2009
2361
Informatics approaches to understanding TGFbeta pathway regulation.
[19855015] Development 136(22):3729-40 (2009)

2009
2362
Recruitment of polycomb group complexes and their role in the dynamic regulation of cell fate choice.
[19820181] Development 136(21):3531-42 (2009)

2010
2363
Organogenetic tolerance.
[21220963] Organogenesis 6(4):270-5 (2010)

2010
2364
Regulation of cellular chromatin state: Insights from quiescence and differentiation.
[20592864] Organogenesis 6(1):37-47 (2010)

2005
2365
Review of awakening agents.
[15825541] Can J Neurol Sci 32(1):4-17 (2005)

2009
2366
The molecular and cellular biology of enhanced cognition.
[19153576] Nat Rev Neurosci 10(2):126-40 (2009)

2007
2367
Femtosecond quantum control of molecular dynamics in the condensed phase.
[17508081] Phys Chem Chem Phys 9(20):2470-97 (2007)

2007
2368
Circular and linear dichroism of proteins.
[17464384] Phys Chem Chem Phys 9(17):2020-35 (2007)

2007
2369
Luminescent chemosensors based on semiconductor quantum dots.
[17464385] Phys Chem Chem Phys 9(17):2036-43 (2007)

2007
2370
Reaction products in mass spectrometry elucidated with infrared spectroscopy.
[17637973] Phys Chem Chem Phys 9(29):3804-17 (2007)

2007
2371
Voids, generic van der Waals equation of state, and transport coefficients of liquids.
[18046466] Phys Chem Chem Phys 9(47):6171-86 (2007)

2007
2372
Fluorescence correlation spectroscopy using quantum dots: advances, challenges and opportunities.
[17431516] Phys Chem Chem Phys 9(16):1870-80 (2007)

2008
2373
Tunneling splitting and decay of metastable states in polyatomic molecules: invariant instanton theory.
[18309393] Phys Chem Chem Phys 10(10):1374-93 (2008)

2008
2374
Physical electrochemistry of nanostructured devices.
[18075682] Phys Chem Chem Phys 10(1):49-72 (2008)

2008
2375
Single molecule magnets: from thin films to nano-patterns.
[18231680] Phys Chem Chem Phys 10(6):784-93 (2008)

2005
2376
The scanned nanopipette: a new tool for high resolution bioimaging and controlled deposition of biomolecules.
[16189604] Phys Chem Chem Phys 7(15):2859-66 (2005)

2009
2377
Simulation of DNA catenanes.
[20145800] Phys Chem Chem Phys 11(45):10543-52 (2009)

2006
2378
Reexamination of ionospheric chemistry: high temperature kinetics, internal energy dependences, unusual isomers, and corrections.
[16738710] Phys Chem Chem Phys 8(22):2557-71 (2006)

2006
2379
Advances in methods and algorithms in a modern quantum chemistry program package.
[16902710] Phys Chem Chem Phys 8(27):3172-91 (2006)

2008
2380
Bridging the gap between protein carboxyl methylation and phospholipid methylation to understand glucose-stimulated insulin secretion from the pancreatic beta cell.
[17662254] Biochem Pharmacol 75(2):335-45 (2008)

2008
2381
Glutamatergic substrates of drug addiction and alcoholism.
[17706608] Biochem Pharmacol 75(1):218-65 (2008)

2008
2382
Sensitive and selective tumor imaging with novel and highly activatable fluorescence probes.
[18187849] Anal Sci 24(1):51-3 (2008)

2010
2383
The lymph node revisited: development, morphology, functioning, and role in triggering primary immune responses.
[20101739] Anat Rec (Hoboken) 293(2):320-37 (2010)

2009
2384
Function of sirtuins in biological tissues.
[19301279] Anat Rec (Hoboken) 292(4):536-43 (2009)

2008
2385
Liver perfusion in sepsis, septic shock, and multiorgan failure.
[18484618] Anat Rec (Hoboken) 291(6):714-20 (2008)

2009
2386
Cellular mechanisms of central nervous system repair by natural autoreactive monoclonal antibodies.
[20008649] Arch Neurol 66(12):1456-9 (2009)

2009
2387
The mirror neuron system.
[19433654] Arch Neurol 66(5):557-60 (2009)

2007
2388
From broken to old: DNA damage, IGF1 endocrine suppression and aging.
[17481965] DNA Repair (Amst) 6(9):1386-90 (2007)

2008
2389
Do all of the neurologic diseases in patients with DNA repair gene mutations result from the accumulation of DNA damage?
[18339586] DNA Repair (Amst) 7(6):834-48 (2008)

2010
2390
Bayes factors in complex genetics.
[20179745] Eur J Hum Genet 18(7):746-50 (2010)

2007
2391
Implication of abnormal epigenetic patterns for human diseases.
[17047674] Eur J Hum Genet 15(1):10-7 (2007)

2009
2392
The enhanced hypercalcemic response to 20-epi-1,25-dihydroxyvitamin D3 results from a selective and prolonged induction of intestinal calcium-regulating genes.
[19423758] Endocrinology 150(8):3448-56 (2009)

2005
2393
The selectivity filter of the cation channel TRPM4.
[15845551] J Biol Chem 280(24):22899-906 (2005)

2003
2394
Mg2+-dependent gating and strong inward rectification of the cation channel TRPV6.
[12601087] J Gen Physiol 121(3):245-60 (2003)

2008
2395
Lithocholic acid derivatives act as selective vitamin D receptor modulators without inducing hypercalcemia.
[18180267] J Lipid Res 49(4):763-72 (2008)

2007
2396
Perspectives on mechanisms of gene regulation by 1,25-dihydroxyvitamin D3 and its receptor.
[17223545] J Steroid Biochem Mol Biol 103(3-5):389-95 (2007)

2009
2397
Tamoxifen inhibits TRPV6 activity via estrogen receptor-independent pathways in TRPV6-expressing MCF-7 breast cancer cells.
[19996302] Mol Cancer Res 7(12):2000-10 (2009)

2005
2398
Large-scale in silico and microarray-based identification of direct 1,25-dihydroxyvitamin D3 target genes.
[16002434] Mol Endocrinol 19(11):2685-95 (2005)

2009
2399
TRPV4-dependent dilation of peripheral resistance arteries influences arterial pressure.
[19617407] Am J Physiol Heart Circ Physiol 297(3):H1096-102 (2009)

2009
2400
Do distinct populations of dorsal root ganglion neurons account for the sensory peptidergic innervation of the kidney?
[19692481] Am J Physiol Renal Physiol 297(5):F1427-34 (2009)

2012
2401
Tissue transglutaminase inhibits the TRPV5-dependent calcium transport in an N-glycosylation-dependent manner.
[21952826] Cell Mol Life Sci 69(6):981-92 (2012)

2009
2402
Store-operated Ca2+ channels and microdomains of Ca2+ in liver cells.
[19196257] Clin Exp Pharmacol Physiol 36(1):77-83 (2009)

2009
2403
Altered central TRPV4 expression and lipid raft association related to inappropriate vasopressin secretion in cirrhotic rats.
[19091909] Am J Physiol Regul Integr Comp Physiol 296(2):R454-66 (2009)

2010
2404
Atomic force microscopy reveals the alternating subunit arrangement of the TRPP2-TRPV4 heterotetramer.
[20682256] Biophys J 99(3):790-7 (2010)

2005
2405
TRPV4 forms a novel Ca2+ signaling complex with ryanodine receptors and BKCa channels.
[16269659] Circ Res 97(12):1270-9 (2005)

2008
2406
Calcium elevation in mouse pancreatic beta cells evoked by extracellular human islet amyloid polypeptide involves activation of the mechanosensitive ion channel TRPV4.
[18751967] Diabetologia 51(12):2252-62 (2008)

2009
2407
Caveolae, caveolin and control of vascular tone: nitric oxide (NO) and endothelium derived hyperpolarizing factor (EDHF) regulation.
[20083858] J Physiol Pharmacol 60 Suppl 4():105-9 (2009)

2007
2408
Loss of Bardet Biedl syndrome proteins causes defects in peripheral sensory innervation and function.
[17959775] Proc Natl Acad Sci U S A 104(44):17524-9 (2007)

2004
2409
Cell swelling, heat, and chemical agonists use distinct pathways for the activation of the cation channel TRPV4.
[14691263] Proc Natl Acad Sci U S A 101(1):396-401 (2004)

2003
2410
Abnormal osmotic regulation in trpv4-/- mice.
[14581612] Proc Natl Acad Sci U S A 100(23):13698-703 (2003)

2006
2411
Ca2+ channels and pulmonary endothelial permeability: insights from study of intact lung and chronic pulmonary hypertension.
[17085430] Microcirculation 13(8):725-39 (2006)

2009
2412
HuR and TTP: two RNA binding proteins that deliver message from the 3' end.
[19327732] Gastroenterology 136(5):1495-8 (2009)

2008
2413
Silencing a killer among us: ethanol impairs immune surveillance of activated stellate cells by natural killer cells.
[18166364] Gastroenterology 134(1):351-3 (2008)

2008
2414
Genomic and epigenetic instability in colorectal cancer pathogenesis.
[18773902] Gastroenterology 135(4):1079-99 (2008)

2006
2415
Erotomania revisited: thirty-four years later.
[16749657] J Natl Med Assoc 98(5):787-93 (2006)

2005
2416
A case of systemic malignant atrophic papulosis (KÃ¶hlmeier-Degos' disease).
[15779511] J Natl Med Assoc 97(3):421-5 (2005)

2008
2417
Exceptional longevity in men: modifiable factors associated with survival and function to age 90 years.
[18268169] Arch Intern Med 168(3):284-90 (2008)

2008
2418
Radiotherapy for management of skin cancers in fibrodysplasia ossificans progressiva: a case report and review of the literature.
[18417900] J Cancer Res Ther 4(1):37-8 (2008)

2008
2419
An overview on applications of optical spectroscopy in cervical cancers.
[18417899] J Cancer Res Ther 4(1):26-36 (2008)

2007
2420
Defect of alveolar regeneration in pulmonary emphysema: role of lung fibroblasts.
[18268920] Int J Chron Obstruct Pulmon Dis 2(4):463-9 (2007)

2009
2421
Implications of bacterial biofilms in chronic rhinosinusitis.
[20191203] Braz J Infect Dis 13(3):232-5 (2009)

2005
2422
Sphingolipids in infectious diseases.
[15973004] Jpn J Infect Dis 58(3):131-48 (2005)

2010
2423
Aminoglycoside-induced mutation suppression (stop codon readthrough) as a therapeutic strategy for Duchenne muscular dystrophy.
[21179598] Ther Adv Neurol Disord 3(6):379-89 (2010)

2010
2424
A preclinical trial of sialic acid metabolites on distal myopathy with rimmed vacuoles/hereditary inclusion body myopathy, a sugar-deficient myopathy: a review.
[21179605] Ther Adv Neurol Disord 3(2):127-35 (2010)

2008
2425
Therapeutic advances and future prospects in immune-mediated inflammatory myopathies.
[21180574] Ther Adv Neurol Disord 1(3):157-66 (2008)

2006
2426
Neurochemistry of the nucleus accumbens and its relevance to depression and antidepressant action in rodents.
[18654637] Curr Neuropharmacol 4(4):277-91 (2006)

2009
2427
Hypocretin/Orexin neuropeptides: participation in the control of sleep-wakefulness cycle and energy homeostasis.
[19721817] Curr Neuropharmacol 7(1):50-9 (2009)

2007
2428
The neurobiological bases for development of pharmacological treatments of aggressive disorders.
[18615178] Curr Neuropharmacol 5(2):135-47 (2007)

2008
2429
Clearing the brain's cobwebs: the role of autophagy in neuroprotection.
[19305790] Curr Neuropharmacol 6(2):97-101 (2008)

2006
2430

PDZ domains at excitatory synapses: potential molecular targets for persistent pain treatment.
[18615145] Curr Neuropharmacol 4(3):217-23 (2006)

2011
2431

Biomarkers in development of psychotropic drugs.
[21842620] Dialogues Clin Neurosci 13(2):225-34 (2011)

2010
2432

Emergent processes in cognitive-emotional interactions.
[21319489] Dialogues Clin Neurosci 12(4):433-48 (2010)

2010
2433

Neurocircuitry of the nicotinic cholinergic system.
[21319492] Dialogues Clin Neurosci 12(4):463-70 (2010)

2010
2434

Human intelligence and brain networks.
[21319494] Dialogues Clin Neurosci 12(4):489-501 (2010)

2010
2435

Compulsive hoarding: current controversies and new directions.
[20623927] Dialogues Clin Neurosci 12(2):233-40 (2010)

2010
2436

Convergence of amyloid-beta and tau pathologies on mitochondria in vivo.
[20217279] Mol Neurobiol 41(2-3):107-14 (2010)

2010
2437

Microglia activation and anti-inflammatory regulation in Alzheimer's disease.
[20195797] Mol Neurobiol 41(2-3):115-28 (2010)

2010
2438

Targeting NADPH oxidase and phospholipases A2 in Alzheimer's disease.
[20195796] Mol Neurobiol 41(2-3):73-86 (2010)

2010
2439

Reperfusion and neurovascular dysfunction in stroke: from basic mechanisms to potential strategies for neuroprotection.
[20157789] Mol Neurobiol 41(2-3):172-9 (2010)

2010
2440

The pathogenic implication of abnormal interaction between apolipoprotein E isoforms, amyloid-beta peptides, and sulfatides in Alzheimer's disease.
[20052565] Mol Neurobiol 41(2-3):97-106 (2010)

2010
2441

"Where, O death, is thy sting?" A brief review of apoptosis biology.
[20552413] Mol Neurobiol 42(1):4-9 (2010)

2010
2442

The roles of the dystrophin-associated glycoprotein complex at the synapse.
[19899002] Mol Neurobiol 41(1):1-21 (2010)

2009
2443

The molecular architecture of ribbon presynaptic terminals.
[19253034] Mol Neurobiol 39(2):130-48 (2009)

2009
2444

Revisiting the stimulus-secretion coupling in the adrenal medulla: role of gap junction-mediated intercellular communication.
[19444654] Mol Neurobiol 40(1):87-100 (2009)

2004
2445

Discovering endophenotypes for major depression.
[15213704] Neuropsychopharmacology 29(10):1765-81 (2004)

2010
2446

The episodic memory system: neurocircuitry and disorders.
[19776728] Neuropsychopharmacology 35(1):86-104 (2010)

2010
2447

Human and rodent homologies in action control: corticostriatal determinants of goal-directed and habitual action.
[19776734] Neuropsychopharmacology 35(1):48-69 (2010)

2010
2448

Normal development of brain circuits.
[19794405] Neuropsychopharmacology 35(1):147-68 (2010)

2010　The reward circuit: linking primate anatomy and human imaging.
2449　[19812543] Neuropsychopharmacology 35(1):4-26 (2010)

2010　Probing compulsive and impulsive behaviors, from animal models to endophenotypes: a narrative
2450　review.
　　　[19940844] Neuropsychopharmacology 35(3):591-604 (2010)

2010　Cortico-Basal Ganglia reward network: microcircuitry.
2451　[19675534] Neuropsychopharmacology 35(1):27-47 (2010)

2010　Neurocircuitry of mood disorders.
2452　[19693001] Neuropsychopharmacology 35(1):192-216 (2010)

2010　Phasic vs sustained fear in rats and humans: role of the extended amygdala in fear vs anxiety.
2453　[19693004] Neuropsychopharmacology 35(1):105-35 (2010)

2010　Neurocircuitry of addiction.
2454　[19710631] Neuropsychopharmacology 35(1):217-38 (2010)

2010　Attention-deficit/hyperactivity disorder and attention networks.
2455　[19759528] Neuropsychopharmacology 35(1):278-300 (2010)

2006　VNS therapy in treatment-resistant depression: clinical evidence and putative neurobiological
2456　mechanisms.
　　　[16641939] Neuropsychopharmacology 31(7):1345-55 (2006)

2010　Brain reward circuitry beyond the mesolimbic dopamine system: a neurobiological theory.
2457　[20149820] Neurosci Biobehav Rev 35(2):129-50 (2010)

2009　Cognitive control mechanisms, emotion and memory: a neural perspective with implications for
2458　psychopathology.
　　　[18948135] Neurosci Biobehav Rev 33(5):613-30 (2009)

2009　The anterior insula in autism: under-connected and under-examined.
2459　[19538989] Neurosci Biobehav Rev 33(8):1198-203 (2009)

2008　How do the basal ganglia contribute to categorization? Their roles in generalization, response
2460　selection, and learning via feedback.
　　　[17919725] Neurosci Biobehav Rev 32(2):265-78 (2008)

2007　A key role for corticotropin-releasing factor in alcohol dependence.
2461　[17629579] Trends Neurosci 30(8):399-406 (2007)

2009　The hippocampal rate code: anatomy, physiology and theory.
2462　[19406485] Trends Neurosci 32(6):329-38 (2009)

2008　Axonal growth therapeutics: regeneration or sprouting or plasticity?
2463　[18395807] Trends Neurosci 31(5):215-20 (2008)

2008　Limbic and cortical information processing in the nucleus accumbens.
2464　[18786735] Trends Neurosci 31(11):552-8 (2008)

2009　Neocortical neurogenesis: morphogenetic gradients and beyond.
2465　[19635637] Trends Neurosci 32(8):443-50 (2009)

2011　The inflammasomes: molecular effectors of host resistance against bacterial, viral, parasitic, and
2466　fungal infections.
　　　[21716947] Front Microbiol 2(-):15 (2011)

2010　Mammalian MicroRNAs: Post-Transcriptional Gene Regulation in RNA Virus Infection and
2467　Therapeutic Applications.

[21607080] Front Microbiol 1(-):108 (2010)

2009
2468
Diphosphoinositol polyphosphates: metabolic messengers?
[19439500] Mol Pharmacol 76(2):236-52 (2009)

2009
2469
Siglecs as targets for therapy in immune-cell-mediated disease.
[19359050] Trends Pharmacol Sci 30(5):240-8 (2009)

2011
2470
Antibody-based therapeutics to watch in 2011.
[21051951] MAbs 3(1):76-99 (2011)

2010
2471
Structural insights into G-quadruplexes: towards new anticancer drugs.
[20563318] Future Med Chem 2(4):619-46 (2010)

2010
2472
Insulin-like growth factor-I regulation of immune function: a potential therapeutic target in autoimmune diseases?
[20392809] Pharmacol Rev 62(2):199-236 (2010)

2010
2473
Targeting intermediary metabolism in the hypothalamus as a mechanism to regulate appetite.
[20392806] Pharmacol Rev 62(2):237-64 (2010)

2010
2474
Seven transmembrane receptors as shapeshifting proteins: the impact of allosteric modulation and functional selectivity on new drug discovery.
[20392808] Pharmacol Rev 62(2):265-304 (2010)

2010
2475
Xenobiotic, bile acid, and cholesterol transporters: function and regulation.
[20103563] Pharmacol Rev 62(1):1-96 (2010)

2010
2476
Oxidation of the endogenous cannabinoid arachidonoyl ethanolamide by the cytochrome P450 monooxygenases: physiological and pharmacological implications.
[20133390] Pharmacol Rev 62(1):136-54 (2010)

2007
2477
5-HT receptor regulation of neurotransmitter release.
[18160701] Pharmacol Rev 59(4):360-417 (2007)

2011
2478
Polycomb group proteins are key regulators of keratinocyte function.
[21085188] J Invest Dermatol 131(2):295-301 (2011)

2010
2479
Small is beautiful: insulin-like growth factors and their role in growth, development, and cancer.
[20975071] J Clin Oncol 28(33):4985-95 (2010)

2010
2480
Coprescription of tamoxifen and medications that inhibit CYP2D6.
[20439629] J Clin Oncol 28(16):2768-76 (2010)

2009
2481
American society of clinical oncology clinical practice guideline update on the use of pharmacologic interventions including tamoxifen, raloxifene, and aromatase inhibition for breast cancer risk reduction.
[19470930] J Clin Oncol 27(19):3235-58 (2009)

2010
2482
The clinical potential of microRNAs.
[20925959] J Hematol Oncol 3(-):37 (2010)

2009
2483
Radiation-induced bystander signalling in cancer therapy.
[19377507] Nat Rev Cancer 9(5):351-60 (2009)

2010
2484
Clinical relevance of microparticles from platelets and megakaryocytes.
[20739880] Curr Opin Hematol 17(6):578-84 (2010)

2010
2485
Erythropoietin receptor response circuits.
[20173635] Curr Opin Hematol 17(3):169-76 (2010)

| 2010 | Growth differentiation factor 15 in erythroid health and disease. |
| 2486 | [20182355] Curr Opin Hematol 17(3):184-90 (2010) |

2010 **Growth differentiation factor 15 in erythroid health and disease.**
2486 [20182355] Curr Opin Hematol 17(3):184-90 (2010)

2010 **Recent developments and complexities in neutrophil transmigration.**
2487 [19864945] Curr Opin Hematol 17(1):9-17 (2010)

2009 **Cell adhesion and signaling networks in brain neurovascular units.**
2488 [19318941] Curr Opin Hematol 16(3):209-14 (2009)

2008 **The platelet release reaction: just when you thought platelet secretion was simple.**
2489 [18695380] Curr Opin Hematol 15(5):537-41 (2008)

2009 **WHIM syndrome: congenital immune deficiency disease.**
2490 [19057201] Curr Opin Hematol 16(1):20-6 (2009)

2009 **Giant cell formation and function.**
2491 [19057205] Curr Opin Hematol 16(1):53-7 (2009)

2011 **Cancer screening in the United States, 2011: A review of current American Cancer Society guidelines and issues in cancer screening.**
2492 [21205832] CA Cancer J Clin 61(1):8-30 (2011)

2010 **Isocitrate dehydrogenase 1 and 2 mutations in cancer: alterations at a crossroads of cellular metabolism.**
2493 [20513808] J Natl Cancer Inst 102(13):932-41 (2010)

2010 **Overdiagnosis in cancer.**
2494 [20413742] J Natl Cancer Inst 102(9):605-13 (2010)

2006 **Leptin resistance and obesity.**
2495 [17021377] Obesity (Silver Spring) 14 Suppl 5(-):254S-258S (2006)

2003 **Stereological tools in biomedical research.**
2496 [14605681] An Acad Bras Cienc 75(4):469-86 (2003)

2008 **Radiopharmaceuticals drug interactions: a critical review.**
2497 [19039490] An Acad Bras Cienc 80(4):665-75 (2008)

2007 **Chemical carcinogenesis.**
2498 [18066431] An Acad Bras Cienc 79(4):593-616 (2007)

2007 **Rhodnius prolixus Malpighian tubules and control of diuresis by neurohormones.**
2499 [17401478] An Acad Bras Cienc 79(1):87-95 (2007)

2005 **Bacillus subtilis as a tool for vaccine development: from antigen factories to delivery vectors.**
2500 [15692682] An Acad Bras Cienc 77(1):113-24 (2005)

2009 **Current relevance of fungal and trypanosomatid glycolipids and sphingolipids: studies defining structures conspicuously absent in mammals.**
2501 [19722017] An Acad Bras Cienc 81(3):477-88 (2009)

2009 **The use of Fluorescence Resonance Energy Transfer (FRET) peptides for measurement of clinically important proteolytic enzymes.**
2502 [19722010] An Acad Bras Cienc 81(3):381-92 (2009)

2006 **Secretory organelles of pathogenic protozoa.**
2503 [16710566] An Acad Bras Cienc 78(2):271-91 (2006)

2011 **Primary vascular tumors of bone: a spectrum of entities?**
2504 [21904630] Int J Clin Exp Pathol 4(6):541-51 (2011)

2010 Molecular classification of soft tissue sarcomas and its clinical applications.
2505 [20490332] Int J Clin Exp Pathol 3(4):416-28 (2010)

2010 Glanzmann's thrombasthenia: report of a case and review of the literature.
2506 [20490335] Int J Clin Exp Pathol 3(4):443-7 (2010)

2010 Autoimmune pancreatitis and IgG4-related systemic diseases.
2507 [20606730] Int J Clin Exp Pathol 3(5):491-504 (2010)

2009 Epigenetics and epigenetic alterations in pancreatic cancer.
2508 [19158989] Int J Clin Exp Pathol 2(4):310-26 (2009)

2009 FoxP3: a life beyond regulatory T cells.
2509 [19079616] Int J Clin Exp Pathol 2(3):205-10 (2009)

2009 High-grade prostatic intraepithelial neoplasia of the prostate: the precursor lesion of prostate
2510 cancer.
[19158990] Int J Clin Exp Pathol 2(4):327-38 (2009)

2009 Neuropathology of non-Alzheimer degenerative disorders.
2511 [19918325] Int J Clin Exp Pathol 3(1):1-23 (2009)

2008 Fibrosing cholestatic hepatitis: clinicopathologic spectrum, diagnosis and pathogenesis.
2512 [18787628] Int J Clin Exp Pathol 1(5):396-402 (2008)

2008 Thymic stromal lymphopoietin (TSLP) as a bridge between infection and atopy.
2513 [18787616] Int J Clin Exp Pathol 1(4):325-30 (2008)

2008 Immunohistochemistry for assessment of pulmonary and pleural neoplasms: a review and update.
2514 [18784820] Int J Clin Exp Pathol 1(1):19-31 (2008)

2008 Tissue transglutaminase, protein cross-linking and Alzheimer's disease: review and views.
2515 [18784819] Int J Clin Exp Pathol 1(1):5-18 (2008)

2008 Genetic neuropathology of Parkinson's disease.
2516 [18784814] Int J Clin Exp Pathol 1(3):217-31 (2008)

2009 HMGB1, an innate alarmin, in the pathogenesis of type 1 diabetes.
2517 [19918326] Int J Clin Exp Pathol 3(1):24-38 (2009)

2011 A new Web-based medical tool for assessment and prevention of comprehensive cardiovascular risk.
2518 [21445280] Ther Clin Risk Manag 7(-):59-68 (2011)

2007 Clinical studies with oral lipid based formulations of poorly soluble compounds.
2519 [18472981] Ther Clin Risk Manag 3(4):591-604 (2007)

2011 Pulmonary thromboendarterectomy for chronic thromboembolic pulmonary hypertension : a
2520 systematic review.
[21881372] Ann Thorac Cardiovasc Surg 17(5):435-45 (2011)

2008 Reexpansion pulmonary edema.
2521 [18818568] Ann Thorac Cardiovasc Surg 14(4):205-9 (2008)

2010 Sleeve lobectomy: current indications and future directions.
2522 [21030916] Ann Thorac Cardiovasc Surg 16(5):310-8 (2010)

2007 Utility of the aortic fenestration technique in the management of acute aortic dissections.
2523 [17954985] Ann Thorac Cardiovasc Surg 13(5):296-300 (2007)

2007
2524

Surgical treatment of infected intralobar pulmonary sequestration: a collective review of patients older than 50 years reported in the literature.
[17954990] Ann Thorac Cardiovasc Surg 13(5):331-4 (2007)

2009
2525

Left ventricular reconstruction with or without mitral annuloplasty.
[19597391] Ann Thorac Cardiovasc Surg 15(3):165-70 (2009)

2006
2526

Surgically removed thoracolithiasis: report of two cases.
[16977300] Ann Thorac Cardiovasc Surg 12(4):279-82 (2006)

2010
2527

The Brugada ECG pattern: a marker of channelopathy, structural heart disease, or neither? Toward a unifying mechanism of the Brugada syndrome.
[20551422] Circ Arrhythm Electrophysiol 3(3):283-90 (2010)

2010
2528

Amiodarone versus procainamide for the acute treatment of recurrent supraventricular tachycardia in pediatric patients.
[20194798] Circ Arrhythm Electrophysiol 3(2):134-40 (2010)

2010
2529

The pathophysiologic basis of fractionated and complex electrograms and the impact of recording techniques on their detection and interpretation.
[20407105] Circ Arrhythm Electrophysiol 3(2):204-13 (2010)

2010
2530

Chest compressions cause recurrence of ventricular fibrillation after the first successful conversion by defibrillation in out-of-hospital cardiac arrest.
[20042768] Circ Arrhythm Electrophysiol 3(1):72-8 (2010)

2010
2531

Phase mapping of cardiac fibrillation.
[20160178] Circ Arrhythm Electrophysiol 3(1):105-14 (2010)

2009
2532

Applications of cardiac magnetic resonance in electrophysiology.
[19808444] Circ Arrhythm Electrophysiol 2(1):63-71 (2009)

2009
2533

P wave indices: current status and future directions in epidemiology, clinical, and research applications.
[19808445] Circ Arrhythm Electrophysiol 2(1):72-9 (2009)

2009
2534

The modulated dispersion hypothesis confirmed in humans.
[19808452] Circ Arrhythm Electrophysiol 2(2):100-1 (2009)

2009
2535

Long-term outcomes after catheter ablation of cavo-tricuspid isthmus dependent atrial flutter: a meta-analysis.
[19808495] Circ Arrhythm Electrophysiol 2(4):393-401 (2009)

2009
2536

Supravalvular arrhythmia: identifying and ablating the substrate.
[19808482] Circ Arrhythm Electrophysiol 2(3):316-26 (2009)

2009
2537

New pharmacological agents for arrhythmias.
[19843928] Circ Arrhythm Electrophysiol 2(5):588-97 (2009)

2008
2538

Cryoglobulinaemia: clinical and laboratory perspectives.
[18239245] Hong Kong Med J 14(1):55-9 (2008)

2010
2539

Hypothalamic mechanisms in cachexia.
[20346963] Physiol Behav 100(5):478-89 (2010)

2010
2540

Excess dietary salt intake alters the excitability of central sympathetic networks.
[20434471] Physiol Behav 100(5):519-24 (2010)

2010
2541

The neurohormonal regulation of energy intake in relation to bariatric surgery for obesity.
[20452367] Physiol Behav 100(5):549-59 (2010)

2010 **Estrogen action: a historic perspective on the implications of considering alternative approaches.**
2542   [19737574] Physiol Behav 99(2):151-62 (2010)

2008 **Salt craving: the psychobiology of pathogenic sodium intake.**
2543   [18514747] Physiol Behav 94(5):709-21 (2008)

2008 **Molecular and neural mediators of leptin action.**
2544   [18501391] Physiol Behav 94(5):637-42 (2008)

2008 **De-stabilization of the positive vago-vagal reflex in bulimia nervosa.**
2545   [18191425] Physiol Behav 94(1):136-53 (2008)

2008 **An insight into the biochemistry of inborn errors of metabolism for a clinical neurologist.**
2546   [19893643] Ann Indian Acad Neurol 11(2):68-81 (2008)

2009 **Portomesenteric venous thrombosis after laparoscopic surgery: a systematic literature review.**
2547   [19528384] Arch Surg 144(6):520-6 (2009)

2009 **Application of the International Germ Cell Consensus Classification to the Nova Scotia population of patients with germ cell tumours.**
2548   [19424465] Can Urol Assoc J 3(2):120-4 (2009)

2011 **Signs in chest imaging.**
2549   [20669122] Diagn Interv Radiol 17(1):18-29 (2011)

2011 **Congenital thoracic arterial anomalies in adults: a CT overview.**
2550   [21975665] Diagn Interv Radiol 17(4):352-62 (2011)

2011 **Dual-energy CT revisited with multidetector CT: review of principles and clinical applications.**
2551   [20945292] Diagn Interv Radiol 17(3):181-94 (2011)

2011 **MRI for acute neurologic complications in end-stage renal disease patients on hemodialysis.**
2552   [20683820] Diagn Interv Radiol 17(2):112-7 (2011)

2010 **Percutaneous aspiration thrombectomy in the treatment of lower extremity thromboembolic occlusions.**
2553   [20044798] Diagn Interv Radiol 16(1):79-83 (2010)

2008 **Angiographic signs in specific vasculitides.**
2554   [18814139] Diagn Interv Radiol 14(3):159-62 (2008)

2011 **Involvement of the immune system in idiosyncratic drug reactions.**
2555   [21084762] Drug Metab Pharmacokinet 26(1):47-59 (2011)

2005 **Possible involvement of singlet oxygen species as multiple oxidants in p450 catalytic reactions.**
2556   [15770070] Drug Metab Pharmacokinet 20(1):1-13 (2005)

2010 **Prediction of severe adverse drug reactions using pharmacogenetic biomarkers.**
2557   [20460818] Drug Metab Pharmacokinet 25(2):122-33 (2010)

2010 **Modulation of UDP-glucuronosyltransferase activity by endogenous compounds.**
2558   [20460819] Drug Metab Pharmacokinet 25(2):134-48 (2010)

2010 **Drug interaction studies on new drug applications: current situations and regulatory views in Japan.**
2559   [20208385] Drug Metab Pharmacokinet 25(1):3-15 (2010)

2010 **Theoretical considerations on quantitative prediction of drug-drug interactions.**
2560   [20208388] Drug Metab Pharmacokinet 25(1):48-61 (2010)

2010 **Ongoing challenges in drug interaction safety: from exposure to pharmacogenomics.**
2561 [20208389] Drug Metab Pharmacokinet 25(1):62-71 (2010)

2010 **Emerging new technology: QSAR analysis and MO Calculation to characterize interactions of protein**
2562 **kinase inhibitors with the human ABC transporter, ABCG2 (BCRP).**
[20208390] Drug Metab Pharmacokinet 25(1):72-83 (2010)

2007 **Microdosing for reduction of the time and resources for drug development.**
2563 [17965515] Drug Metab Pharmacokinet 22(5):327 (2007)

2007 **Targeted delivery systems of small interfering RNA by systemic administration.**
2564 [17603214] Drug Metab Pharmacokinet 22(3):142-51 (2007)

2009 **The versatile MHC class I-related FcRn protects IgG and albumin from degradation: implications for**
2565 **development of new diagnostics and therapeutics.**
[19745559] Drug Metab Pharmacokinet 24(4):318-32 (2009)

2008 **Organic cation transporters and their pharmacokinetic and pharmacodynamic consequences.**
2566 [18762711] Drug Metab Pharmacokinet 23(4):243-53 (2008)

2010 **Sulf-2: an extracellular modulator of cell signaling and a cancer target candidate.**
2567 [20629619] Expert Opin Ther Targets 14(9):935-49 (2010)

2008 **Chromatin-modifying enzymes as therapeutic targets--Part 2.**
2568 [18851700] Expert Opin Ther Targets 12(11):1457-67 (2008)

2008 **Chromatin-modifying enzymes as therapeutic targets--Part 1.**
2569 [18781828] Expert Opin Ther Targets 12(10):1301-12 (2008)

2008 **The paraventricular nucleus of the hypothalamus - a potential target for integrative treatment of**
2570 **autonomic dysfunction.**
[18479218] Expert Opin Ther Targets 12(6):717-27 (2008)

2009 **Targeting SGK1 in diabetes.**
2571 [19764891] Expert Opin Ther Targets 13(11):1303-11 (2009)

2010 **Phyllanthus niruri as a promising alternative treatment for nephrolithiasis.**
2572 [21176271] Int Braz J Urol 36(6):657-64; discussion 664 (2010)

2008 **Difficult male urethral catheterization: a review of different approaches.**
2573 [18778491] Int Braz J Urol 34(4):401-11; discussion 412 (2008)

2010 **Ureteral endometriosis: a rare and underdiagnosed cause of kidney dysfunction.**
2574 [19887828] Nephron Clin Pract 114(2):c89-93 (2010)

2011 **Hydrodynamic gene delivery and its applications in pharmaceutical research.**
2575 [21191634] Pharm Res 28(4):694-701 (2011)

2008 **Click chemistry, a powerful tool for pharmaceutical sciences.**
2576 [18509602] Pharm Res 25(10):2216-30 (2008)

2010 **Embolization in trauma: principles and techniques.**
2577 [21359011] Semin Intervent Radiol 27(1):14-28 (2010)

2004 **Transcatheter arterial embolization in the trauma patient: a review.**
2578 [21331105] Semin Intervent Radiol 21(1):11-22 (2004)

2008 **Obstetric and gynecologic emergencies: a review of indications and interventional techniques.**
2579 [21326575] Semin Intervent Radiol 25(4):337-46 (2008)

2008 **An overview of embolic agents.**
2580   [21326511] Semin Intervent Radiol 25(3):204-15 (2008)

2011 **Increased heart rate and atherosclerosis: potential implications of ivabradine therapy.**
2581   [21526046] World J Cardiol 3(4):101-4 (2011)

2011 **Future easy and physiological cardiac pacing.**
2582   [21286216] World J Cardiol 3(1):32-9 (2011)

2011 **Advantages and disadvantages of biodegradable platforms in drug eluting stents.**
2583   [21499496] World J Cardiol 3(3):84-92 (2011)

2011 **Differential diagnosis of tachycardia with a typical left bundle branch block morphology.**
2584   [21666813] World J Cardiol 3(5):127-34 (2011)

2010 **Management and therapy of vasovagal syncope: A review.**
2585   [21160608] World J Cardiol 2(10):308-15 (2010)

2010 **Use of the impedance threshold device in cardiopulmonary resuscitation.**
2586   [21160680] World J Cardiol 2(2):19-26 (2010)

2010 **Speckle tracking echocardiography: A new approach to myocardial function.**
2587   [21160657] World J Cardiol 2(1):1-5 (2010)

2011 **Intrinsic and extrinsic regulation of innate immune receptors.**
2588   [21488180] Yonsei Med J 52(3):379-92 (2011)

2010 **Intrinsic cellular defenses against virus infection by antiviral type I interferon.**
2589   [20046508] Yonsei Med J 51(1):9-17 (2010)

2003 **Gordius worm found in a three year old girl's vomitus.**
2590   [12833600] Yonsei Med J 44(3):557-60 (2003)

2008 **Roles of embryonic and adult lymphoid tissue inducer cells in primary and secondary lymphoid tissues.**
2591   [18581582] Yonsei Med J 49(3):352-6 (2008)

2011 **Glutamine supplementation.**
2592   [21906372] Ann Intensive Care 1(1):25 (2011)

2011 **Microcirculatory alterations: potential mechanisms and implications for therapy.**
2593   [21906380] Ann Intensive Care 1(1):27 (2011)

2011 **Understanding urine output in critically ill patients.**
2594   [21906341] Ann Intensive Care 1(1):13 (2011)

2010 **Narrative review: the systemic capillary leak syndrome.**
2595   [20643990] Ann Intern Med 153(2):90-8 (2010)

2009 **Narrative review: the emerging clinical implications of the role of aldosterone in the metabolic syndrome and resistant hypertension.**
2596   [19487712] Ann Intern Med 150(11):776-83 (2009)

2010 **Peritoneal transport testing.**
2597   [20540028] J Nephrol 23(6):633-47 (2010)

2010 **Evaluation of glomerular filtration rate and of albuminuria/proteinuria.**
2598   [20213606] J Nephrol 23(2):125-32 (2010)

2009 Sympathetic activation in cardiovascular and renal disease.
2599   [19384835] J Nephrol 22(2):190-5 (2009)

2009 Disturbances of glomerular hemodynamics: a risk factor determing progression of glomerular
2600   diseases?
       [19384836] J Nephrol 22(2):196-202 (2009)

2009 Xenobiotic kidney organogenesis: a new avenue for renal transplantation.
2601   [19557707] J Nephrol 22(3):312-7 (2009)

2011 Monoclonal B-cell lymphocytosis: a brief review for general clinicians.
2602   [21755252] Sao Paulo Med J 129(3):171-5 (2011)

2009 Oral drugs for hypertensive urgencies: systematic review and meta-analysis.
2603   [20512292] Sao Paulo Med J 127(6):366-72 (2009)

2009 Hepatopulmonary syndrome: an update.
2604   [20011928] Sao Paulo Med J 127(4):223-30 (2009)

2010 Tnk1/Kos1: a novel tumor suppressor.
2605   [20697568] Trans Am Clin Climatol Assoc 121(-):281-92; discussion 292-3 (2010)

2009 How do kidney cells adapt to survive in hypertonic inner medulla?
2606   [19768191] Trans Am Clin Climatol Assoc 120(-):389-401 (2009)

2009 The inherited autoinflammatory syndrome: a decade of discovery.
2607   [19768193] Trans Am Clin Climatol Assoc 120(-):413-8 (2009)

2009 Ageing and the glomerular filtration rate: truths and consequences.
2608   [19768194] Trans Am Clin Climatol Assoc 120(-):419-28 (2009)

2009 The role of circulating mesenchymal progenitor cells, fibrocytes, in promoting pulmonary fibrosis.
2609   [19768162] Trans Am Clin Climatol Assoc 120(-):49-59 (2009)

2011 Avoidable deaths in the first four years of life among children in the 2004 Pelotas (Brazil) birth
2610   cohort study.
       [21789412] Cad Saude Publica 27 Suppl 2(-):S185-97 (2011)

2009 Environment, interactions between Trypanosoma cruzi and its host, and health.
2611   [19287864] Cad Saude Publica 25 Suppl 1(-):S32-44 (2009)

2005 Specific therapy based on the genotype and cellular mechanism in inherited cardiac arrhythmias.
2612   Long QT syndrome and Brugada syndrome.
       [15892662] Curr Pharm Des 11(12):1561-72 (2005)

2010 Echinoderms: potential model systems for studies on muscle regeneration.
2613   [20041824] Curr Pharm Des 16(8):942-55 (2010)

2009 Nicotinamide phosphoribosyltransferase (Nampt): a link between NAD biology, metabolism, and
2614   diseases.
       [19149599] Curr Pharm Des 15(1):20-8 (2009)

2009 The importance of NAD in multiple sclerosis.
2615   [19149604] Curr Pharm Des 15(1):64-99 (2009)

2009 Developmental and pathogenic mechanisms of basement membrane assembly.
2616   [19355968] Curr Pharm Des 15(12):1277-94 (2009)

2009 Lactoferrin as a natural immune modulator.
2617   [19519436] Curr Pharm Des 15(17):1956-73 (2009)

2010	**Practical aspects of insulin pen devices.**
2618	[20513316] J Diabetes Sci Technol 4(3):522-31 (2010)

2010	**Evolution of diabetes insulin delivery devices.**
2619	[20513314] J Diabetes Sci Technol 4(3):505-13 (2010)

2008	**Use of continuous subcutaneous insulin infusion (insulin pump) therapy in the hospital: a review of one institution's experience.**
2620	[19885284] J Diabetes Sci Technol 2(6):948-62 (2008)

2011	**Optical imaging in vivo with a focus on paediatric disease: technical progress, current preclinical and clinical applications and future perspectives.**
2621	[21221568] Pediatr Radiol 41(2):161-75 (2011)

2011	**Hepatobiliary and pancreatic imaging in children-techniques and an overview of non-neoplastic disease entities.**
2622	[20967540] Pediatr Radiol 41(1):55-75 (2011)

2010	**Diffusion imaging and tractography of congenital brain malformations.**
2623	[19937239] Pediatr Radiol 40(1):59-67 (2010)

2009	**Radiation-sensitive genetically susceptible pediatric sub-populations.**
2624	[19083227] Pediatr Radiol 39 Suppl 1(-):S27-31 (2009)

2008	**Malfunctioning central venous catheters in children: a diagnostic approach.**
2625	[17932667] Pediatr Radiol 38(4):363-78, quiz 486-7 (2008)

2004	**Diagnostic imaging of diffuse infiltrative disease of the lung.**
2626	[14872104] Respiration 71(1):4-19 (2004)

2004	**Interstitial lung disease induced by drugs and radiation.**
2627	[15316202] Respiration 71(4):301-26 (2004)

2004	**Rare infiltrative lung diseases: a challenge for clinicians.**
2628	[15467318] Respiration 71(5):431-43 (2004)

2003	**Newly diagnosed chronic obstructive pulmonary disease. Clinical features and distribution of the novel stages of the Global Initiative for Obstructive Lung Disease.**
2629	[12584394] Respiration 70(1):67-75 (2003)

2010	**Sodium channel molecular conformations and antiarrhythmic drug affinity.**
2630	[20685573] Trends Cardiovasc Med 20(1):16-21 (2010)

2007	**Rebuilding the coronary vasculature: hedgehog as a new candidate for pharmacologic revascularization.**
2631	[17418368] Trends Cardiovasc Med 17(3):77-83 (2007)

2008	**Neutrophils as sources of extracellular nucleotides: functional consequences at the vascular interface.**
2632	[18436149] Trends Cardiovasc Med 18(3):103-7 (2008)

2009	**Aldehyde dehydrogenase 2 in cardiac protection: a new therapeutic target?**
2633	[20005475] Trends Cardiovasc Med 19(5):158-64 (2009)

2011	**Management of pulmonary embolism with rheolytic thrombectomy.**
2634	[22059183] Can Respir J 18(4):e52-8 (2011)

2005	**New methodology in biomedical science: methodological errors in classical science.**
2635	[15687745] Medicina (Kaunas) 41(1):7-16 (2005)

2008
2636

Genetically modified organisms: do the benefits outweigh the risks?
[18344661] Medicina (Kaunas) 44(2):87-99 (2008)

2011
2637

Enhancement of solute removal in a hollow-fiber hemodialyzer by mechanical vibration.
[21242675] Blood Purif 31(4):227-34 (2011)

2010
2638

Mechanical ventilation and the kidney.
[19923815] Blood Purif 29(1):52-68 (2010)

2010
2639

Modern classification of acute kidney injury.
[20130395] Blood Purif 29(3):300-7 (2010)

2009
2640

Role of vasopressin and vasopressin receptor antagonists in type I cardiorenal syndrome.
[19169014] Blood Purif 27(1):28-32 (2009)

2011
2641

PARP inhibitors: its role in treatment of cancer.
[21718592] Chin J Cancer 30(7):463-71 (2011)

2011
2642

Single-nucleotide polymorphisms among microRNA: big effects on cancer.
[21627860] Chin J Cancer 30(6):381-91 (2011)

2010
2643

Clinical practice. Protein-losing enteropathy in children.
[20571826] Eur J Pediatr 169(10):1179-85 (2010)

2011
2644

Educational paper: Primary immunodeficiencies in children: a diagnostic challenge.
[21170549] Eur J Pediatr 170(2):169-77 (2011)

2011
2645

Educational paper: primary antibody deficiencies.
[21544519] Eur J Pediatr 170(6):693-702 (2011)

2011
2646

Educational paper: screening in cancer predisposition syndromes: guidelines for the general pediatrician.
[21210147] Eur J Pediatr 170(3):285-94 (2011)

2011
2647

Educational paper: syndromic forms of primary immunodeficiency.
[21337117] Eur J Pediatr 170(3):295-308 (2011)

2011
2648

Educational paper. The expanding clinical and immunological spectrum of severe combined immunodeficiency.
[21479529] Eur J Pediatr 170(5):561-71 (2011)

2009
2649

Molecular genetic analysis of podocyte genes in focal segmental glomerulosclerosis--a review.
[19562370] Eur J Pediatr 168(11):1291-304 (2009)

2006
2650

A review of the biochemistry, metabolism and clinical benefits of thiamin(e) and its derivatives.
[16550223] Evid Based Complement Alternat Med 3(1):49-59 (2006)

2010
2651

Intraoperative detection of gamma emissions using K-alpha X-ray fluorescence.
[20583879] Expert Rev Med Devices 7(4):431-4 (2010)

2011
2652

The future of the artificial kidney: moving towards wearable and miniaturized devices.
[21270908] Nefrologia 31(1):9-16 (2011)

2010
2653

The lectin-like oxidized low-density lipoprotein receptor-1 and its soluble form: cardiovascular implications.
[20009416] J Atheroscler Thromb 17(4):317-31 (2010)

2010
2654

Protein-phospholipid interactions in blood clotting.
[20129649] Thromb Res 125 Suppl 1(-):S23-5 (2010)

2008   **Role of tissue factor disulfides and lipid rafts in signaling.**
2655   [18691492] Thromb Res 122 Suppl 1(-):S14-8 (2008)

2011   **A promising diagnostic method: Terahertz pulsed imaging and spectroscopy.**
2656   [21512652] World J Radiol 3(3):55-65 (2011)

2010   **Pleiotropic effects of intravascular haemolysis on vascular homeostasis.**
2657   [19958359] Br J Haematol 148(5):690-701 (2010)

2009   **Update in understanding common variable immunodeficiency disorders (CVIDs) and the management of patients with these conditions.**
2658   [19344423] Br J Haematol 145(6):709-27 (2009)

2008   **Developing idiotype vaccines for lymphoma: from preclinical studies to phase III clinical trials.**
2659   [18422783] Br J Haematol 142(2):179-91 (2008)

2010   **Toxicities of the thrombopoietic growth factors.**
2660   [20620441] Semin Hematol 47(3):289-98 (2010)

2010   **Neonatal thrombocytopenia and megakaryocytopoiesis.**
2661   [20620440] Semin Hematol 47(3):281-8 (2010)

2010   **Platelet formation.**
2662   [20620432] Semin Hematol 47(3):220-6 (2010)

2010   **Megakaryopoiesis.**
2663   [20620431] Semin Hematol 47(3):212-9 (2010)

2010   **Antigenic modulation and rituximab resistance.**
2664   [20350659] Semin Hematol 47(2):124-32 (2010)

2009   **Pathobiology of secondary immune thrombocytopenia.**
2665   [19245930] Semin Hematol 46(1 Suppl 2):S2-14 (2009)

2007   **The structure and function of the Rh antigen complex.**
2666   [17198846] Semin Hematol 44(1):42-50 (2007)

2009   **Emerging treatments for multiple myeloma: beyond immunomodulatory drugs and bortezomib.**
2667   [19389500] Semin Hematol 46(2):166-75 (2009)

2008   **Factor VIIa interaction with tissue factor and endothelial cell protein C receptor on cell surfaces.**
2668   [18544419] Semin Hematol 45(2 Suppl 1):S21-4 (2008)

2008   **Radioimmunotherapy-based conditioning regimens for stem cell transplantation.**
2669   [18381107] Semin Hematol 45(2):118-25 (2008)

2009   **Iron sequestration and anemia of inflammation.**
2670   [19786207] Semin Hematol 46(4):387-93 (2009)

2009   **Animal models of anemia of inflammation.**
2671   [19786203] Semin Hematol 46(4):351-7 (2009)

2007   **The chronic myeloproliferative disorders and mutation of JAK2: Dameshek's 54 year old speculation comes of age.**
2672   [17336249] Best Pract Res Clin Haematol 20(1):5-12 (2007)

2007   **The stem cell niche in health and leukemic disease.**
2673   [17336251] Best Pract Res Clin Haematol 20(1):19-27 (2007)

2010   **Immunomodulation for inhibitors in hemophilia A: the important role of Treg cells.**
2674   [20976115] Expert Rev Hematol 3(4):469-83 (2010)

2011   **SALL4: finally an answer to the problem of expansion of hematopoietic stem cells?**
2675   [21939414] Expert Rev Hematol 4(5):479-81 (2011)

2010   **Antibodies to serine proteases in the antiphospholipid syndrome.**
2676   [20425533] Curr Rheumatol Rep 12(1):45-52 (2010)

2010   **Computational methods for de novo protein design and its applications to the human immunodeficiency virus 1, purine nucleoside phosphorylase, ubiquitin specific protease 7, and histone demethylases.**
2677   [20210752] Curr Drug Targets 11(3):264-78 (2010)

2008   **Thrombospondin and apoptosis: molecular mechanisms and use for design of complementation treatments.**
2678   [18855619] Curr Drug Targets 9(10):851-62 (2008)

2008   **Enhancing cardiovascular dynamics by inhibition of thrombospondin-1/CD47 signaling.**
2679   [18855617] Curr Drug Targets 9(10):833-41 (2008)

2010   **Erythropoietin for infants with hypoxic-ischemic encephalopathy.**
2680   [20090525] Curr Opin Pediatr 22(2):139-45 (2010)

2011   **Internet pathways in suicidality: a review of the evidence.**
2681   [22073021] Int J Environ Res Public Health 8(10):3938-52 (2011)

2008   **Genome-wide association studies: progress and potential for drug discovery and development.**
2682   [18274536] Nat Rev Drug Discov 7(3):221-30 (2008)

2008   **The TWEAK-Fn14 cytokine-receptor axis: discovery, biology and therapeutic targeting.**
2683   [18404150] Nat Rev Drug Discov 7(5):411-25 (2008)

2009   **Immunomodulatory effects of deacetylase inhibitors: therapeutic targeting of FOXP3+ regulatory T cells.**
2684   [19855427] Nat Rev Drug Discov 8(12):969-81 (2009)

2003   **Cerebral mass lesion due to cytomegalovirus in a patient with AIDS: case report and literature review.**
2685   [14762635] Rev Inst Med Trop Sao Paulo 45(6):333-7 (2003)

2010   **Gastrointestinal and hepatic manifestations of primary immune deficiency diseases.**
2686   [20339173] Saudi J Gastroenterol 16(2):66-74 (2010)

2011   **Rapid analysis of pharmacology for infectious diseases.**
2687   [21401504] Curr Top Med Chem 11(10):1292-300 (2011)

2010   **Emerging methods for ensemble-based virtual screening.**
2688   [19929833] Curr Top Med Chem 10(1):3-13 (2010)

2009   **ITK inhibitors in inflammation and immune-mediated disorders.**
2689   [19689375] Curr Top Med Chem 9(8):690-703 (2009)

2009   **The pilot phase of the NIH Chemical Genomics Center.**
2690   [19807664] Curr Top Med Chem 9(13):1181-93 (2009)

2011   **Contact endoscopy as a novel technique in the detection and diagnosis of mucosal lesions in the head and neck: a brief review.**
2691   [21209710] J Oncol 2011(-):196302 (2011)

2011
2692
Autoantibodies to tailor-made panels of tumor-associated antigens in breast carcinoma.
[21423545] J Oncol 2011(-):982425 (2011)

2011
2693
Lipid mediators and human leukemic blasts.
[20953410] J Oncol 2011(-):- (2011)

2011
2694
Intracellular cAMP signaling by soluble adenylyl cyclase.
[21490586] Kidney Int 79(12):1277-88 (2011)

2009
2695
A dietary non-human sialic acid may facilitate hemolytic-uremic syndrome.
[19387473] Kidney Int 76(2):140-4 (2009)

2011
2696
Free Fatty Acid receptors and their physiological role in metabolic regulation.
[22129861] Yakugaku Zasshi 131(12):1683-9 (2011)

2007
2697
Insulin resistance as a membrane microdomain disorder.
[17409686] Yakugaku Zasshi 127(4):579-86 (2007)

2010
2698
Review of catumaxomab in the treatment of malignant ascites.
[21188120] Cancer Manag Res 2(-):283-6 (2010)

2009
2699
Extracorporeal photopheresis-induced immune tolerance: a focus on modulation of antigen-presenting cells and induction of regulatory T cells by apoptotic cells.
[19444106] Curr Opin Organ Transplant 14(4):338-43 (2009)

2011
2700
A review of the role of solar ultraviolet-B irradiance and vitamin D in reducing risk of dental caries.
[22110779] Dermatoendocrinol 3(3):193-8 (2011)

2008
2701
IGF-1 receptor inhibitors in clinical trials--early lessons.
[19023648] J Mammary Gland Biol Neoplasia 13(4):471-83 (2008)

2009
2702
Macrophages in breast cancer: do involution macrophages account for the poor prognosis of pregnancy-associated breast cancer?
[19350209] J Mammary Gland Biol Neoplasia 14(2):145-57 (2009)

2009
2703
Transforming growth factor-(beta)s and mammary gland involution; functional roles and implications for cancer progression.
[19396528] J Mammary Gland Biol Neoplasia 14(2):131-44 (2009)

2011
2704
Robotic-assisted transoral removal of a bilateral floor of mouth ranulas.
[21767364] World J Surg Oncol 9(-):78 (2011)

2010
2705
Predictive and prognostic molecular markers for cancer medicine.
[21789130] Ther Adv Med Oncol 2(2):125-48 (2010)

2010
2706
Crucial role of CGI-58/alpha/beta hydrolase domain-containing protein 5 in lipid metabolism.
[20190389] Biol Pharm Bull 33(3):342-5 (2010)

2009
2707
Oligovascular signaling in white matter stroke.
[19801821] Biol Pharm Bull 32(10):1639-44 (2009)

2011
2708
Fibrocytes and the tissue niche in lung repair.
[21658209] Respir Res 12(-):76 (2011)

2008
2709
Mass spectrometric quantification of amino acid oxidation products identifies oxidative mechanisms of diabetic end-organ damage.
[18752069] Rev Endocr Metab Disord 9(4):275-87 (2008)

2011
2710
Left Atrial Appendage Closure in Atrial Fibrillation: A World without Anticoagulation?
[21559225] Cardiol Res Pract 2011(-):752808 (2011)

2010
2711   Fingertip digital thermal monitoring: a fingerprint for cardiovascular disease?
         [20012695] Int J Cardiovasc Imaging 26(2):249-52 (2010)

2011
2712   Advanced treatments in non-clear renal cell carcinoma.
         [21404194] Urol J 8(1):1-11 (2011)

2002
2713   Maxillary removal and reinsertion in pediatric patients.
         [11784250] Arch Otolaryngol Head Neck Surg 128(1):29-34 (2002)

2008
2714   Caveolin-1, transforming growth factor-beta receptor internalization, and the pathogenesis of
         systemic sclerosis.
         [18949888] Curr Opin Rheumatol 20(6):713-9 (2008)

2010
2715   Neutrophil gelatinase-associated lipocalin and hepcidin: what do they have in common and is there
         a potential interaction?
         [20502037] Kidney Blood Press Res 33(2):157-65 (2010)

2011
2716   Glucan-immunostimulant, adjuvant, potential drug.
         [21603320] World J Clin Oncol 2(2):115-9 (2011)

2011
2717   Role of optical spectroscopy using endogenous contrasts in clinical cancer diagnosis.
         [21603314] World J Clin Oncol 2(1):50-63 (2011)

2011
2718   Optical mammography: Diffuse optical imaging of breast cancer.
         [21603315] World J Clin Oncol 2(1):64-72 (2011)

2008
2719   The PAT family of lipid droplet proteins in heart and vascular cells.
         [18959832] Curr Hypertens Rep 10(6):461-6 (2008)

2011
2720   MicroRNAs in lipid metabolism.
         [21178770] Curr Opin Lipidol 22(2):86-92 (2011)

2007
2721   GPIHBP1: an endothelial cell molecule important for the lipolytic processing of chylomicrons.
         [17620854] Curr Opin Lipidol 18(4):389-96 (2007)

2009
2722   GPIHBP1 and lipolysis: an update.
         [19369870] Curr Opin Lipidol 20(3):211-6 (2009)

2008
2723   Emigration of monocyte-derived cells to lymph nodes during resolution of inflammation and its
         failure in atherosclerosis.
         [18769227] Curr Opin Lipidol 19(5):462-8 (2008)

2007
2724   Kinase packing defects as drug targets.
         [17993409] Drug Discov Today 12(21-22):917-23 (2007)

2008
2725   Biosynthesis, degradation and pharmacological importance of the fatty acid amides.
         [18598910] Drug Discov Today 13(13-14):558-68 (2008)

2008
2726   The application of FAST-NMR for the identification of novel drug discovery targets.
         [18275915] Drug Discov Today 13(3-4):172-9 (2008)

2011
2727   Anticancer targets in the glycolytic metabolism of tumors: a comprehensive review.
         [21904528] Front Pharmacol 2(-):49 (2011)

2011
2728   From understanding cellular function to novel drug discovery: the role of planar patch-clamp array
         chip technology.
         [22007170] Front Pharmacol 2(-):51 (2011)

2011
2729   TRP Channels as Sensors and Signal Integrators of Redox Status Changes.
         [22016736] Front Pharmacol 2(-):58 (2011)

2010 **The CCN proteins: important signaling mediators in stem cell differentiation and tumorigenesis.**
2730 [20376786] Histol Histopathol 25(6):795-806 (2010)

2010 **Gli-similar (Glis) KrÃ¼ppel-like zinc finger proteins: insights into their physiological functions and**
2731 **critical roles in neonatal diabetes and cystic renal disease.**
      [20865670] Histol Histopathol 25(11):1481-96 (2010)

2010 **Specification of arterial, venous, and lymphatic endothelial cells during embryonic development.**
2732 [20238301] Histol Histopathol 25(5):637-46 (2010)

2010 **The early endosome: a busy sorting station for proteins at the crossroads.**
2733 [19924646] Histol Histopathol 25(1):99-112 (2010)

2010 **Heme-dependent and independent soluble guanylate cyclase activators and vasodilation.**
2734 [20571429] J Cardiovasc Pharmacol 56(3):229-33 (2010)

2010 **Targeting epoxides for organ damage in hypertension.**
2735 [20531214] J Cardiovasc Pharmacol 56(4):329-35 (2010)

2010 **20-hydroxyeicosatetraeonic acid: a new target for the treatment of hypertension.**
2736 [20930591] J Cardiovasc Pharmacol 56(4):336-44 (2010)

2005 **A modular theory of autoimmunity.**
2737 [16237273] Keio J Med 54(3):121-6 (2005)

2008 **Paraneoplastic syndromes of the CNS.**
2738 [18339348] Lancet Neurol 7(4):327-40 (2008)

2010 **Endoscopic hemostasis techniques for upper gastrointestinal hemorrhage: A review.**
2739 [21160691] World J Gastrointest Endosc 2(2):54-60 (2010)

2010 **Mallory-Denk body pathogenesis revisited.**
2740 [21161012] World J Hepatol 2(8):295-301 (2010)

2010 **Fucosylation and gastrointestinal cancer.**
2741 [21160988] World J Hepatol 2(4):151-61 (2010)

2006 **Three-dimensional atlas of lymph node topography based on the visible human data set.**
2742 [16783763] Anat Rec B New Anat 289(3):98-111 (2006)

2011 **The use of an implantable Doppler flow probe in kidney transplantation: first report in the literature.**
2743 [21453229] Exp Clin Transplant 9(2):118-20 (2011)

2009 **The counteradhesive proteins, thrombospondin 1 and SPARC/osteonectin, open the tyrosine**
2744 **phosphorylation-responsive paracellular pathway in pulmonary vascular endothelia.**
      [18952113] Microvasc Res 77(1):13-20 (2009)

2009 **Regulation of vascular permeability by sphingosine 1-phosphate.**
2745 [18973762] Microvasc Res 77(1):39-45 (2009)

2009 **The actin cytoskeleton in endothelial cell phenotypes.**
2746 [19028505] Microvasc Res 77(1):53-63 (2009)

2008 **Molecular mechanisms of preeclampsia.**
2747 [17553534] Microvasc Res 75(1):1-8 (2008)

2008 **The role of cytoskeleton in the regulation of vascular endothelial barrier function.**
2748 [18657550] Microvasc Res 76(3):202-7 (2008)

2011
2749
Cytoplasmic overexpression of CD95L in esophageal adenocarcinoma cells overcomes resistance to CD95-mediated apoptosis.
[21390183] Neoplasia 13(3):198-205 (2011)

2010
2750
Nmp4/CIZ: road block at the intersection of PTH and load.
[19766748] Bone 46(2):259-66 (2010)

2011
2751
MVP and vaults: a role in the radiation response.
[22040803] Radiat Oncol 6(-):148 (2011)

2010
2752
Molecular regulation of vasculogenic mimicry in tumors and potential tumor-target therapy.
[21160860] World J Gastrointest Surg 2(4):117-27 (2010)

2010
2753
Non-invasive assessment of barrier integrity and function of the human gut.
[21160852] World J Gastrointest Surg 2(3):61-9 (2010)

2006
2754
Evacuation of hematomas using liposuction technology: Technique and literature review.
[19554234] Can J Plast Surg 14(1):51-2 (2006)

2010
2755
Out cold: biochemical regulation of mammalian hibernation - a mini-review.
[19602865] Gerontology 56(2):220-30 (2010)

2010
2756
P2X(7) receptor at the heart of disease.
[20981163] Hippokratia 14(3):155-63 (2010)

2010
2757
The effects of hemodynamic force on embryonic development.
[20374481] Microcirculation 17(3):164-78 (2010)

2010
2758
Tumor microvasculature and microenvironment: novel insights through intravital imaging in pre-clinical models.
[20374484] Microcirculation 17(3):206-25 (2010)

2008
2759
Theoretical models of microvascular oxygen transport to tissue.
[18608981] Microcirculation 15(8):795-811 (2008)

2008
2760
Systems biology of vascular endothelial growth factors.
[18608994] Microcirculation 15(8):715-38 (2008)

2008
2761
Computational and mathematical modeling of angiogenesis.
[18720228] Microcirculation 15(8):739-51 (2008)

2008
2762
Modeling structural adaptation of microcirculation.
[18802843] Microcirculation 15(8):753-64 (2008)

2008
2763
The role of theoretical modeling in microcirculation research.
[18946803] Microcirculation 15(8):693-8 (2008)

2008
2764
Theoretical models for regulation of blood flow.
[18951240] Microcirculation 15(8):765-75 (2008)

2009
2765
The myoendothelial junction: breaking through the matrix?
[19330678] Microcirculation 16(4):307-22 (2009)

2008
2766
Nonepileptic motor phenomena in the neonate.
[19436521] Paediatr Child Health 13(8):680-4 (2008)

2009
2767
Guidelines for paediatric emergency equipment and supplies for a physician's office.
[20592979] Paediatr Child Health 14(6):402-4 (2009)

2007
2768
Heme as a magnificent molecule with multiple missions: heme determines its own fate and governs cellular homeostasis.
[17785948] Tohoku J Exp Med 213(1):1-16 (2007)

2008
2769
Anosognosia for amnesia as a clue to understand the nature of dementia.
[18577843] Tohoku J Exp Med 215(2):141-7 (2008)

2010
2770
SDH-related pheochromocytoma and paraganglioma.
[20833333] Best Pract Res Clin Endocrinol Metab 24(3):415-24 (2010)

2010
2771
Metabolic consequences of intermittent hypoxia: relevance to obstructive sleep apnea.
[21112030] Best Pract Res Clin Endocrinol Metab 24(5):843-51 (2010)

2010
2772
Obstructive sleep apnea: role in the risk and severity of diabetes.
[21112020] Best Pract Res Clin Endocrinol Metab 24(5):703-15 (2010)

2007
2773
The MCT8 thyroid hormone transporter and Allan-Herndon-Dudley syndrome.
[17574010] Best Pract Res Clin Endocrinol Metab 21(2):307-21 (2007)

2010
2774
Boolean versus ranked querying for biomedical systematic reviews.
[20937152] BMC Med Inform Decis Mak 10(-):58 (2010)

2009
2775
Circulating MicroRNA Signatures of Tumor-Derived Exosomes for Early Diagnosis of Non-Small-Cell Lung Cancer.
[19289365] Clin Lung Cancer 10(1):8-9 (2009)

2011
2776
Inhibitors of Glioma Growth that Reveal the Tumour to the Immune System.
[22084619] Clin Med Insights Oncol 5(-):265-314 (2011)

2009
2777
Dendritic cells in immunotherapy of established cancer: Roles of signals 1, 2, 3 and 4.
[19513941] Curr Opin Investig Drugs 10(6):526-35 (2009)

2010
2778
Irreversible electroporation: a novel image-guided cancer therapy.
[21103304] Gut Liver 4 Suppl 1(-):S99-S104 (2010)

2011
2779
Pathophysiological consequences of hemolysis. Role of cell-free hemoglobin.
[22100795] Postepy Hig Med Dosw (Online) 65(0):627-39 (2011)

2006
2780
Late-phase 3 EAD. A unique mechanism contributing to initiation of atrial fibrillation.
[16606397] Pacing Clin Electrophysiol 29(3):290-5 (2006)

2010
2781
Pathophysiology and clinical implications of cardiac memory.
[20025710] Pacing Clin Electrophysiol 33(3):346-52 (2010)

2010
2782
Anatomy and electrophysiology of the human AV node.
[20180918] Pacing Clin Electrophysiol 33(6):754-62 (2010)

2007
2783
The importance of hormesis to public health.
[17680154] Cien Saude Colet 12(4):955-63 (2007)

2010
2784
Nanotechnology applications in surgical oncology.
[20059343] Annu Rev Med 61(-):359-73 (2010)

2011
2785
New developments in the treatment of hyperammonemia: emerging use of carglumic acid.
[21403788] Int J Gen Med 4(-):21-8 (2011)

2011
2786
Emerging treatment options for short bowel syndrome: potential role of teduglutide.
[22016579] Clin Exp Gastroenterol 4(-):189-96 (2011)

2011
2787
Statistical physics approaches to neuronal network dynamics.
[22002236] Sheng Li Xue Bao 63(5):453-62 (2011)

2008
2788
Recent evidence for activity-dependent initiation of sympathetic sprouting and neuropathic pain.
[18958370] Sheng Li Xue Bao 60(5):617-27 (2008)

2008
2789
A role for uninjured afferents in neuropathic pain.
[18958368] Sheng Li Xue Bao 60(5):605-9 (2008)

2009
2790
Coronary microvascular resistance: methods for its quantification in humans.
[19468781] Basic Res Cardiol 104(5):485-98 (2009)

2010
2791
Clinical trials of pharmacological therapies in acute heart failure syndromes: lessons learned and directions forward.
[20233993] Circ Heart Fail 3(2):314-25 (2010)

2011
2792
Bnip3 as a dual regulator of mitochondrial turnover and cell death in the myocardium.
[21210091] Pediatr Cardiol 32(3):267-74 (2011)

2011
2793
Cardiomyocyte death: insights from molecular and microstructural magnetic resonance imaging.
[21298427] Pediatr Cardiol 32(3):290-6 (2011)

2011
2794
Statin therapy in metabolic syndrome and hypertension post-JUPITER: what is the value of CRP?
[21046291] Curr Atheroscler Rep 13(1):31-42 (2011)

2011
2795
Role of phospholipid transfer protein in high-density lipoprotein- mediated reverse cholesterol transport.
[21365262] Curr Atheroscler Rep 13(3):242-8 (2011)

2011
2796
Role of hepatic lipase and endothelial lipase in high-density lipoprotein-mediated reverse cholesterol transport.
[21424685] Curr Atheroscler Rep 13(3):257-65 (2011)

2010
2797
Mitochondrial pruning by Nix and BNip3: an essential function for cardiac-expressed death factors.
[20559783] J Cardiovasc Transl Res 3(4):374-83 (2010)

2011
2798
Circulating very small embryonic-like stem cells in cardiovascular disease.
[21165781] J Cardiovasc Transl Res 4(2):138-44 (2011)

2010
2799
Injectable materials for the treatment of myocardial infarction and heart failure: the promise of decellularized matrices.
[20632221] J Cardiovasc Transl Res 3(5):478-86 (2010)

2010
2800
Imaging and modeling of myocardial metabolism.
[20559785] J Cardiovasc Transl Res 3(4):384-96 (2010)

2010
2801
Extracorporeal irradiated tumor bone: A reconstruction option in diaphyseal Ewing's sarcomas.
[20924479] Indian J Orthop 44(4):390-6 (2010)

2009
2802
Reparative dentinogenesis induced by mineral trioxide aggregate: a review from the biological and physicochemical points of view.
[20339574] Int J Dent 2009(-):464280 (2009)

2010
2803
ASIA or Shoenfeld's syndrome: a novel autoimmune syndrome?
[21125185] Rev Bras Reumatol 50(5):487-8 (2010)

2011
2804
The clinical impact of bacterial biofilms.
[21485309] Int J Oral Sci 3(2):55-65 (2011)

2010
2805
Lymphangiogenesis, lymphatic endothelial cells and lymphatic metastasis in head and neck cancer-- a review of mechanisms.

[20690413] Int J Oral Sci 2(1):5-14 (2010)

2010
2806
The role of NELL-1, a growth factor associated with craniosynostosis, in promoting bone regeneration.
[20647499] J Dent Res 89(9):865-78 (2010)

2010
2807
Strong nanocomposites with Ca, PO(4), and F release for caries inhibition.
[19948941] J Dent Res 89(1):19-28 (2010)

2010
2808
Extracellular matrix: a gatekeeper in the transition from dormancy to metastatic growth.
[20304630] Eur J Cancer 46(7):1181-8 (2010)

2010
2809
A medicinal chemist's guide to molecular interactions.
[20345171] J Med Chem 53(14):5061-84 (2010)

2011
2810
Organometallic anticancer compounds.
[21077686] J Med Chem 54(1):3-25 (2011)

2010
2811
Pathogenesis of allergic airway inflammation.
[20425513] Curr Allergy Asthma Rep 10(1):39-48 (2010)

2002
2812
Immune-based therapies: a review of clinical endpoints used in trials of selected immunologic agents.
[11819187] HIV Clin Trials 3(1):58-88 (2002)

2011
2813
Towards BioDBcore: a community-defined information specification for biological databases.
[21205783] Database (Oxford) 2011(-):baq027 (2011)

2011
2814
PubMed and beyond: a survey of web tools for searching biomedical literature.
[21245076] Database (Oxford) 2011(-):baq036 (2011)

2008
2815
Glucocorticoids shift arachidonic acid metabolism toward endocannabinoid synthesis: a non-genomic anti-inflammatory switch.
[18295199] Eur J Pharmacol 583(2-3):322-39 (2008)

2003
2816
Sources and significance of plasma levels of catechols and their metabolites in humans.
[12649306] J Pharmacol Exp Ther 305(3):800-11 (2003)

2008
2817
Stratum corneum lipid organization as observed by atomic force, confocal and two-photon excitation fluorescence microscopy.
[19099542] Int J Cosmet Sci 30(6):391-411 (2008)

2008
2818
In vivo reflectance-mode confocal microscopy in clinical dermatology and cosmetology.
[18377626] Int J Cosmet Sci 30(1):1-17 (2008)

2007
2819
Identification of type I interferon-associated inflammation in the pathogenesis of cutaneous lupus erythematosus opens up options for novel therapeutic approaches.
[17437489] Exp Dermatol 16(5):454-63 (2007)

2009
2820
Emergency lateral canthotomy and cantholysis: a simple procedure to preserve vision from sight threatening orbital hemorrhage.
[19739474] J Spec Oper Med 9(3):26-32 (2009)

2007
2821
MELD score, step forward to justice of liver graft allocation in Brazil.
[18060268] Arq Gastroenterol 44(3):187-8 (2007)

2011
2822
Hormesis pervasiveness and its potential implications for pharmaceutical research and development.
[22013400] Dose Response 9(3):377-86 (2011)

2011
2823
Editorial: is airport body-scan radiation a health risk?
[21431083] Dose Response 9(1):1-5 (2011)

2010   **Radiation hormesis: historical perspective and implications for low-dose cancer risk assessment.**
2824   [20585444] Dose Response 8(2):172-91 (2010)

2011   **Reduction of myocardial infarct size by dronedarone in pigs--a pleiotropic action?**
2825   [21544523] Cardiovasc Drugs Ther 25(3):197-201 (2011)

2011   **Cardiac resynchronization therapy in patients with mild heart failure: a systematic review and meta-analysis of randomized controlled trials.**
2826   [21750900] Cardiovasc Drugs Ther 25(4):331-40 (2011)

2009   **Phospholipase A2 biochemistry.**
2827   [18931897] Cardiovasc Drugs Ther 23(1):49-59 (2009)

2010   **The Pathogenesis and treatment of the valvulopathy of aortic stenosis: Beyond the SEAS.**
2828   [20425167] Curr Cardiol Rep 12(2):125-32 (2010)

2010   **The evolution of transcranial laser therapy for acute ischemic stroke, including a pooled analysis of NEST-1 and NEST-2.**
2829   [20425181] Curr Cardiol Rep 12(1):29-33 (2010)

2010   **A meta-analysis of glucose-insulin-potassium therapy for treatment of acute myocardial infarction.**
2830   [20631859] Exp Clin Cardiol 15(2):e20-4 (2010)

2005   **Pathophysiological role of autoantibodies against G-protein-coupled receptors in the cardiovascular system.**
2831   [19641683] Exp Clin Cardiol 10(3):170-2 (2005)

2011   **Chronic ventricular pacing in children: toward prevention of pacing-induced heart disease.**
2832   [21107685] Heart Fail Rev 16(3):305-14 (2011)

2007   **Imaging ventricular fibrillation,**
2833   [17993330] J Electrocardiol 40(6 Suppl):S56-61 (2007)

2007   **Imaging fibrillation/defibrillation in a dish.**
2834   [17993331] J Electrocardiol 40(6 Suppl):S62-5 (2007)

2007   **Eight (or more) kinds of alternans.**
2835   [17993333] J Electrocardiol 40(6 Suppl):S70-4 (2007)

2005   **Is there an overlap between Brugada syndrome and arrhythmogenic right ventricular cardiomyopathy/dysplasia?**
2836   [16003713] J Electrocardiol 38(3):260-3 (2005)

2010   **Ferroportin disease: a systematic meta-analysis of clinical and molecular findings.**
2837   [20691492] J Hepatol 53(5):941-9 (2010)

2008   **Clinical, pathological, and molecular correlates in ferroportin disease: a study of two novel mutations.**
2838   [18713659] J Hepatol 49(4):664-71 (2008)

2009   **Treatment failure in hepatitis C: mechanisms of non-response.**
2839   [19070928] J Hepatol 50(2):412-20 (2009)

2011   **Periostin expression and epithelial-mesenchymal transition in cancer: a review and an update.**
2840   [21997759] Virchows Arch 459(5):465-75 (2011)

2010   **Running GAGs: myxoid matrix in tumor pathology revisited: what's in it for the pathologist?**
2841   [19705152] Virchows Arch 456(2):181-92 (2010)

2010   **Genome-scale approaches to the epigenetics of common human disease.**
2842   [19844740] Virchows Arch 456(1):13-21 (2010)

2003   **Tumor reversion: correction of malignant behavior by microenvironmental cues.**
2843   [14566816] Int J Cancer 107(5):688-95 (2003)

2008   **Optical contrast agents and imaging systems for detection and diagnosis of cancer.**
2844   [18712733] Int J Cancer 123(9):1979-90 (2008)

2009   **Lymphatics in idiopathic pulmonary fibrosis: new insights into an old disease.**
2845   [20143918] Lymphat Res Biol 7(4):197-203 (2009)

2008   **Developmental angiogenesis of the central nervous system.**
2846   [19093790] Lymphat Res Biol 6(3-4):173-80 (2008)

2010   **Emerging roles for multimodal optical imaging in early cancer detection: a global challenge.**
2847   [20218743] Technol Cancer Res Treat 9(2):211-7 (2010)

2003   **Optical systems for in vivo molecular imaging of cancer.**
2848   [14640761] Technol Cancer Res Treat 2(6):491-504 (2003)

2008   **Helical tomotherapy: a fascinating technological concept that has matured into clinical reality.**
2849   [19044319] Technol Cancer Res Treat 7(6):415-6 (2008)

2010   **Advances in pharmacologic stress agents: focus on regadenoson.**
2850   [20724531] J Nucl Med Technol 38(3):163-71 (2010)

2011   **Year in review in Intensive Care Medicine 2010: II. Pneumonia and infections, cardiovascular and**
2851   **haemodynamics, organization, education, haematology, nutrition, ethics and miscellanea.**
    [21225240] Intensive Care Med 37(2):196-213 (2011)

2011   **Year in review in Intensive Care Medicine 2010: I. Acute renal failure, outcome, risk assessment and**
2852   **ICU performance, sepsis, neuro intensive care and experimentals.**
    [21203748] Intensive Care Med 37(1):19-34 (2011)

2011   **Year in review in Intensive Care Medicine 2010: III. ARDS and ALI, mechanical ventilation,**
2853   **noninvasive ventilation, weaning, endotracheal intubation, lung ultrasound and paediatrics.**
    [21290103] Intensive Care Med 37(3):394-410 (2011)

2010   **The use of botulinum toxin as primary or adjunctive treatment for post acne and traumatic scarring.**
2854   [21031067] J Cutan Aesthet Surg 3(2):90-2 (2010)

2006   **X-Ray microanalytical techniques based on synchrotron radiation.**
2855   [16395457] J Environ Monit 8(1):33-42 (2006)

2007   **Aquatic environmental nanoparticles.**
2856   [18049768] J Environ Monit 9(12):1306-16 (2007)

2011   **Biological effects of electromagnetic fields and recently updated safety guidelines for strong static**
2857   **magnetic fields.**
    [21441722] Magn Reson Med Sci 10(1):1-10 (2011)

2006   **Amplification of spatial dispersion of repolarization underlies sudden cardiac death associated with**
2858   **catecholaminergic polymorphic VT, long QT, short QT and Brugada syndromes.**
    [16336513] J Intern Med 259(1):48-58 (2006)

2010   **Type 2 transglutaminase in Huntington's disease: a double-edged sword with clinical potential.**
2859   [20964734] J Intern Med 268(5):419-31 (2010)

2010   **Redox sensing: orthogonal control in cell cycle and apoptosis signalling.**
2860   [20964735] J Intern Med 268(5):432-48 (2010)

2010   **The neurovascular unit in the setting of stroke.**
2861   [20175864] J Intern Med 267(2):156-71 (2010)

| 2009 | **Modulating T-cell homeostasis with IL-7: preclinical and clinical studies.** |
| 2862 | [19623690] J Intern Med 266(2):141-53 (2009) |

| 2010 | **Autophagy: assays and artifacts.** |
| 2863 | [20225337] J Pathol 221(2):117-24 (2010) |

| 2010 | **Autophagy: cellular and molecular mechanisms.** |
| 2864 | [20225336] J Pathol 221(1):3-12 (2010) |

| 2003 | **Pathogenetic mechanisms in usual interstitial pneumonia/idiopathic pulmonary fibrosis.** |
| 2865 | [14595745] J Pathol 201(3):343-54 (2003) |

| 2010 | **The pathobiology of splicing.** |
| 2866 | [19918805] J Pathol 220(2):152-63 (2010) |

| 2008 | **Cellular and molecular mechanisms of fibrosis.** |
| 2867 | [18161745] J Pathol 214(2):199-210 (2008) |

| 2008 | **Macrophage activation by endogenous danger signals.** |
| 2868 | [18161744] J Pathol 214(2):161-78 (2008) |

| 2009 | **Activated macrophages in the tumour microenvironment-dancing to the tune of TLR and NF-kappaB.** |
| 2869 | [19662665] J Pathol 219(2):143-52 (2009) |

| 2010 | **DNA diagnostics: nanotechnology-enhanced electrochemical detection of nucleic acids.** |
| 2870 | [20075759] Pediatr Res 67(5):458-68 (2010) |

| 2008 | **Hamartomatous polyposis syndromes.** |
| 2871 | [18672141] Surg Clin North Am 88(4):779-817, vii (2008) |

| 2007 | **Autonomic innervation and regulation of the immune system (1987-2007).** |
| 2872 | [17467231] Brain Behav Immun 21(6):736-45 (2007) |

| 2008 | **Anti-inflammatory neuropeptides: a new class of endogenous immunoregulatory agents.** |
| 2873 | [18598752] Brain Behav Immun 22(8):1146-51 (2008) |

| 2009 | **Contemporary surgery for obstructive sleep apnea syndrome.** |
| 2874 | [19784401] Clin Exp Otorhinolaryngol 2(3):107-14 (2009) |

| 2009 | **Renal cell therapy and beyond.** |
| 2875 | [20017829] Semin Dial 22(6):603-9 (2009) |

| 2009 | **Clinical interpretation of antinuclear antibody tests in systemic rheumatic diseases.** |
| 2876 | [19277826] Mod Rheumatol 19(3):219-28 (2009) |

| 2008 | **The role of cell death in the pathogenesis of autoimmune disease: HMGB1 and microparticles as intercellular mediators of inflammation.** |
| 2877 | [18418695] Mod Rheumatol 18(4):319-26 (2008) |

| 2011 | **Wallerian degeneration: gaining perspective on inflammatory events after peripheral nerve injury.** |
| 2878 | [21878126] J Neuroinflammation 8(-):110 (2011) |

| 2011 | **Alzheimer's disease - a neurospirochetosis. Analysis of the evidence following Koch's and Hill's criteria.** |
| 2879 | [21816039] J Neuroinflammation 8(-):90 (2011) |

| 2008 | **Potential mechanisms of the human polyomavirus JC in neural oncogenesis.** |
| 2880 | [18648329] J Neuropathol Exp Neurol 67(8):729-40 (2008) |

2008
2881

Update on recent molecular and genetic advances in frontotemporal lobar degeneration.
[18596549] J Neuropathol Exp Neurol 67(7):635-48 (2008)

2009
2882

Temporal lobe sclerosis associated with hippocampal sclerosis in temporal lobe epilepsy: neuropathological features.
[19606061] J Neuropathol Exp Neurol 68(8):928-38 (2009)

2008
2883

DNA damage and repair: relevance to mechanisms of neurodegeneration.
[18431258] J Neuropathol Exp Neurol 67(5):377-87 (2008)

2008
2884

Alzheimer disease pathology as a host response.
[18520771] J Neuropathol Exp Neurol 67(6):523-31 (2008)

2009
2885

Chronic traumatic encephalopathy in athletes: progressive tauopathy after repetitive head injury.
[19535999] J Neuropathol Exp Neurol 68(7):709-35 (2009)

2011
2886

Amyloid in the islets of Langerhans: thoughts and some historical aspects.
[21486192] Ups J Med Sci 116(2):81-9 (2011)

2010
2887

Quantitative proton magnetic resonance spectroscopy and spectroscopic imaging of the brain: a didactic review.
[21613876] Top Magn Reson Imaging 21(2):115-28 (2010)

2005
2888

Magnetic resonance imaging-guided vascular interventions.
[16924170] Top Magn Reson Imaging 16(5):369-81 (2005)

2009
2889

Chronic diarrhea due to excessive bile acid synthesis and not defective ileal transport: a new syndrome of defective fibroblast growth factor 19 release.
[19665580] Clin Gastroenterol Hepatol 7(11):1151-4 (2009)

2012
2890

Tutorial review for understanding of cholangiopathy.
[21994886] Int J Hepatol 2012(-):547840 (2012)

2007
2891

Totect: a new agent for treating anthracycline extravasation.
[17623623] Clin J Oncol Nurs 11(3):387-95 (2007)

2008
2892

Putting evidence into practice: evidence-based interventions for the management of oral mucositis.
[18258584] Clin J Oncol Nurs 12(1):141-52 (2008)

2009
2893

Biological barriers to therapy with antisense and siRNA oligonucleotides.
[19397332] Mol Pharm 6(3):686-95 (2009)

2009
2894

Extracellularly activated nanocarriers: a new paradigm of tumor targeted drug delivery.
[19366234] Mol Pharm 6(4):1041-51 (2009)

2010
2895

N-acetylcysteine in acute pancreatitis.
[21577291] World J Gastrointest Pharmacol Ther 1(1):21-6 (2010)

2010
2896

Hard and soft micro- and nanofabrication: An integrated approach to hydrogel-based biosensing and drug delivery.
[20036310] J Control Release 141(3):303-13 (2010)

2010
2897

The role of GNAS and other imprinted genes in the development of obesity.
[19844212] Int J Obes (Lond) 34(1):6-17 (2010)

2010
2898

Frequency of injury and the ecology of regeneration in marine benthic invertebrates.
[21558216] Integr Comp Biol 50(4):479-93 (2010)

2010
2899

Evolutionary loss of animal regeneration: pattern and process.
[21558220] Integr Comp Biol 50(4):515-27 (2010)

| 2010 | **The peril of the plankton.** |
| 2900 | [21558224] Integr Comp Biol 50(4):552-70 (2010) |

| 2010 | **Variety is the spice of life histories: comparison of intraspecific variability in marine invertebrates.** |
| 2901 | [21558229] Integr Comp Biol 50(4):630-42 (2010) |

| 2010 | **It's about time: divergence, demography, and the evolution of developmental modes in marine invertebrates.** |
| 2902 | [21558230] Integr Comp Biol 50(4):643-61 (2010) |

| 2010 | **Coral-associated bacterial assemblages: current knowledge and the potential for climate-driven impacts.** |
| 2903 | [21558231] Integr Comp Biol 50(4):662-74 (2010) |

| 2009 | **Physiologic measures of sexual function in women: a review.** |
| 2904 | [19046582] Fertil Steril 92(1):19-34 (2009) |

| 2010 | **Antifibrinolytics in liver surgery.** |
| 2905 | [21224964] Indian J Anaesth 54(6):489-95 (2010) |

| 2006 | **Premalignant conditions of bone.** |
| 2906 | [16897210] J Orthop Sci 11(4):412-23 (2006) |

| 2007 | **Circuits formultisensory integration and attentional modulation through the prefrontal cortex and the thalamic reticular nucleus in primates.** |
| 2907 | [18330211] Rev Neurosci 18(6):417-38 (2007) |

| 2008 | **Role of signal transducer and activator of transcription 3 in neuronal survival and regeneration.** |
| 2908 | [19145989] Rev Neurosci 19(4-5):341-61 (2008) |

| 2008 | **Recombinant T cell receptor ligands: immunomodulatory, neuroprotective and neuroregenerative effects suggest application as therapy for multiple sclerosis.** |
| 2909 | [19145988] Rev Neurosci 19(4-5):327-39 (2008) |

| 2010 | **The neuro-ophthalmology of mitochondrial disease.** |
| 2910 | [20471050] Surv Ophthalmol 55(4):299-334 (2010) |

| 2008 | **Diagnostic tools for glaucoma detection and management.** |
| 2911 | [19038620] Surv Ophthalmol 53 Suppl1(-):S17-32 (2008) |

| 2011 | **Clearing the complexity: immune complexes and their treatment in lupus nephritis.** |
| 2912 | [21694945] Int J Nephrol Renovasc Dis 4(-):17-28 (2011) |

| 2010 | **Clinical utility of tolvaptan in the management of hyponatremia in heart failure patients.** |
| 2913 | [21694929] Int J Nephrol Renovasc Dis 3(-):51-60 (2010) |

| 2010 | **Signaling mechanisms in thyroid hormone-induced cardiac hypertrophy.** |
| 2914 | [20005976] Vascul Pharmacol 52(3-4):113-9 (2010) |

| 2010 | **Macrophage cholesteryl ester mobilization and atherosclerosis.** |
| 2915 | [19878739] Vascul Pharmacol 52(1-2):1-10 (2010) |

| 2011 | **Computational models of the pulmonary circulation: Insights and the move towards clinically directed studies.** |
| 2916 | [22034608] Pulm Circ 1(2):224-38 (2011) |

| 2011 | **Diagnosis and assessment of pulmonary vascular disease by Doppler echocardiography.** |
| 2917 | [22034604] Pulm Circ 1(2):160-81 (2011) |

| 2011 | **Acute respiratory distress syndrome: A clinical review.** |
| 2918 | [22034606] Pulm Circ 1(2):192-211 (2011) |

2008
2919

Mechanisms of disease: detrimental adrenergic signaling in acute decompensated heart failure.
[18283305] Nat Clin Pract Cardiovasc Med 5(4):208-18 (2008)

2008
2920

Mechanisms of disease: molecular genetics of arrhythmogenic right ventricular dysplasia/cardiomyopathy.
[18382419] Nat Clin Pract Cardiovasc Med 5(5):258-67 (2008)

www.ingramcontent.com/pod-product-compliance
Lightning Source LLC
Chambersburg PA
CBHW051525170526
45165CB00002B/607